Simply Beautiful

A Beauty Encyclopedia

Rima Soni

Foreword by Vimla Patil

BPI (INDIA) PVT LTD

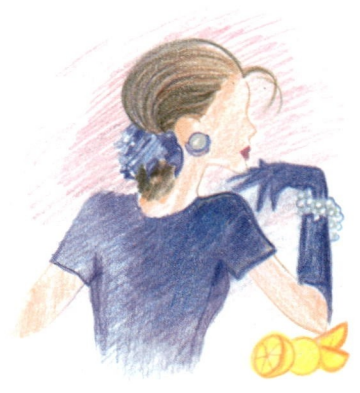

ISBN 81-7693-082-2
©Rima Soni, 2000
©Illustrations Sharmistha Kaushal, 2000

Editor Mridula Maluste
Computer Graphics & Layouts Vicky Sheorey
Cover photograph Boman Irani
Cover design Dhan Cordo
Inside Illustrations Sharmistha Kaushal

Published by
BPI (INDIA) PVT LTD
229/A Krantiveer Rajguru Marg
Girgaon Mumbai 400 004
Phone 385 0661 385 1829   Fax 387 2625
e-mail bpipl@vsnl.com

All rights reserved

Dedicated to my husband Manu and my sons Kunal and Karan. Without their unstinting support, confidence and help, this beauty diary would not have been possible.

A very special thanks to my parents for their sincere love and unending concern for me all these years.

Foreword

BEAUTY IS A WOMAN'S BIRTHRIGHT!

In every age of history, women have constantly, relentlessly, searched for ways to remain young, sensual and beautiful. To be beautiful, decorated and remain attractive to their men was their duty as per many ancient texts. This search first began in their own kitchens and gardens where condiments, spices and herbs provided them with natural beauty aids and remedies for ordinary beauty problems. They used henna, hibiscus, turmeric, cream, spice powders and floral essences to achieve beauty and sensuality. As women realised the importance of beauty and fitness further, their search led them to investigate many therapies such as a aromatherapy, naturopathy, yoga, ayurveda, homeopathy and herbal preparations. Each of these opened ever new doors to the treasure of beauty culture which generations of Indian women used for seeking beauty of face and figure.

In the last century, however, this search further led women to look into products not made from natural resources but from chemicals. Major corporations in the world jumped onto the beauty bandwagon. World-wide brands were built up and sold to women in every country. Exclusive designers like Coco Chanel, Estee Lauder, Yves St.Laurent, and their colleagues from Italy, Britain, France, Germany and the United States made lipsticks, creams, perfumes and a hundred other beauty aids to pamper and spoil women with a promise of ethereal and lasting beauty. Their publicity and marketing strategies were so strong and well designed, that elite women everywhere began to take pride in using exclusive products made by them and even to prove their social status by their choice.

In time, other cheaper brands were launched by multinationals to reach the huge mass of high street shoppers who could not afford designer goods, yet wanted to be as beautiful, as sensual as the celebrities or stars. Naturally, in a market which swallowed beauty related goods like some legendary giant, spurious goods proliferated. Harmful chemicals, allergen-riddled creams and even skin or hair-damaging chemical ingredients were used to make cheap but attractive cosmetics.

In the seventies and eighties, this scary scenario led women to turn with new hope to a back-to-basics lifestyle which spawned herbal products, custom-made or manufactured on a large scale. In England, Anita Roddick made a huge success of her Body Shop chain of outlets, where cosmetics made from pure natural ingredients were sold with awe-inspiring success. If Roddick created a miracle in the West, Shahnaz Husain created an empire from the East by marketing totally herbal cosmetics to meet the needs of beauty conscious women. Today, an incredible variety of beauty products and herbal cosmetics are available the world over and their sale increases in direct proportion to the rising awareness of beauty and fitness among women of all ages.

In India at the present time, this awareness of beauty has reached a crescendo. To begin with Indian women have had total freedom to seek beauty from a vast heritage of beauty for centuries. With beauty contests becoming national events and with Indian women winning international beauty crowns, their awareness and need for beauty has enhanced manifold. This awareness has also reached a new high because of satellite TV which beams into every home attractive lifestyles in which women almost scintillate with beauty and elegance. Thirdly, more and more women are exposed to a glamour-driven world through their education, careers, travel and the advent of multi media events. The result is that beauty has become the credo of Indian women and a serious business for the commercial community. The only difference is that a large number of women now want beauty and fitness as their personal asset or as an asset for commercial success rather than merely to please their men.

In this complex scenario, Rima Soni, a beauty consultant who lives and works in Dubai, has lit a beacon of excitement and hope. She has brought the back-to-basics routine of women 180 degrees around and pointed once again in the direction of the kitchen. She has proved that this gentle heart of every home can provide an answer to every beauty problem a woman can face. Rima has long experience of creating magic potions and mixes from simple ingredients like turmeric, pepper, cream and yoghurt. Now, Simply Beautiful is Rima's offering to women. Her message to them is to participate in the revolution of home beauty which she started some years ago with spectacular success. This book will surely add a spirit of adventure to the lives of all women who will find exploring their kitchens for beauty aids a fun-filled voyage of discovery!

VIMLA PATIL

CONTENTS

1 Introduction

3 Your Food: The Goodness Within

12 The Enemy Within... Your Food?

15 Smoother, Softer Skin

23 Those Tumultuous Teens

31 Say it with your Eyes

34 Occasion-al Beauty

Do your Hands and Legs need a Hand ?

Tone That Body

Facing Wrinkles

Highlight on: Hair

Treat those Problems

Your Questions ... Answered

The Finishing Touch

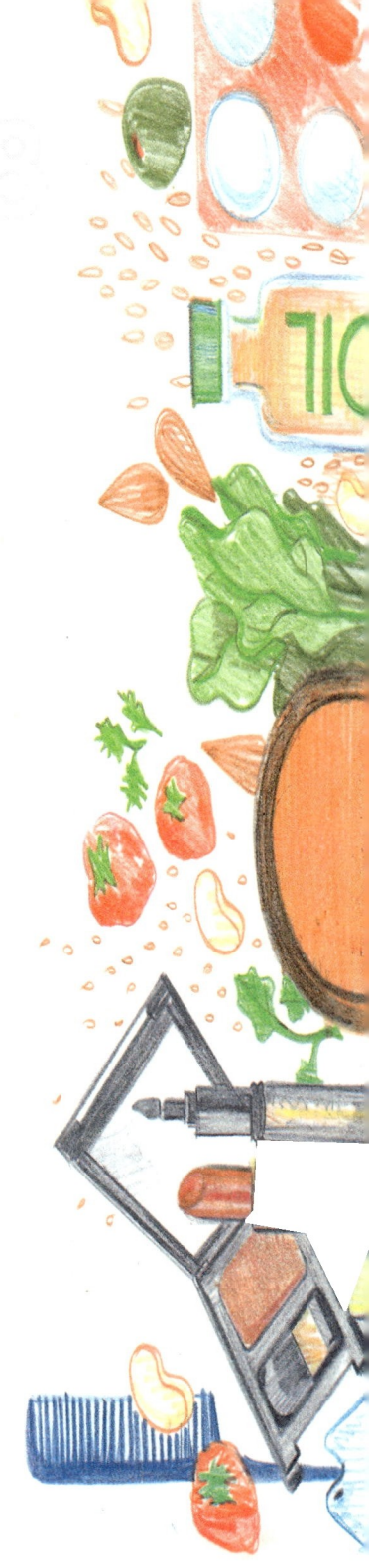

Introduction

How did it all begin? What sparked this lifelong passion? One afternoon, in the year 1978, whilst browsing through some beauty journals, I saw an advertisement for a professional beauty course in London. My eyes twinkled. Within minutes, I was on the phone to my husband. I asked him if he would grant me just one wish ... and of course he agreed! So, I expressed my desire to attend the course.

Within days, I was winging my way to London. Though it was tough being on my own - I'd always led a sheltered, protected life - I enjoyed the months that followed. Situated in the heart of UK, the Beauty school is one of the best in UK. They had a bunch of dedicated and experienced teachers who gave us a thorough, theoretical and practical grounding in 'Aesthetics,' - the study of skin care.

Following my return to Bombay, we were posted to Baghdad. Teeming with ideas from my newly acquired training and restless to put them to immediate use, I began to explore the marketplace. But possibilities were limited as few beauty products or materials were available locally. I was determined - nothing would deter me. Looking around, I realised that I need never have to depend on international beauty care products. I had an amazing range of essentials close at hand, products that would be available in any normal, functioning household. Refrigerators, pantries and backgardens of most homes would have honey, milk, yogurt, almonds, fruits and vegetables. Natural, home products have an edge over supermarket ones: they rarely run out of stock, are easily accessible and within economic reach of almost any housewife.

I began experimenting with different ingredients; studying their food values and effect on various skin types. I became confident that natural kitchen ingredients worked on par with, if not better than commercially prepared beauty care products. In India, it is de rigeur that new born babies be cleansed with emulsions of milk, cream and turmeric instead of soap, as soap is considered harsh on young skin.

We left Baghdad for India end 1979 and I started a small beauty clinic from my Bombay apartment. Discovering that people followed natural beauty therapy or 'kitchen cosmetics' happily, boosted my confidence hugely. Age was no bar-- I experimented on people from 9 to 70. It was a fantastic experience for me. My mother was a great help -- a fund of information. She shared with me a host of beauty remedies that have probably come down the generations. For two years, I must have experimented on over 200 clients. It was great.

1981, and we were on the move again, this time to Dubai. Dubai was and always will be special. It gave me the kind of exposure every professional craves. My husband, Manu was behind my success every inch of the way. I started contributing a beauty column to "Gulf News"; and then got a big break with "Khaleej Times" where, again, I was a regular columnist. I soon, however, ran out of ideas! - a problem that possibly glares most columnists in their face at some time in their careers. My husband, seeing my frustration, suggested I include a question-answer column in the papers. This proved to be a big hit and personally very satisfying as it brought me close to my readers.

This book is very special as I have included a whole range of beauty techniques and treatments I've been following with myself and my clients for ages. It's unique format will enable you to refer to it easily and quickly. You can carry it with you anywhere! Today, with the growing concern over conservation issues, and the movement towards ecologically friendly products, 'Kitchen Cosmetology', I think, is here to stay.

So...next time you have strawberries and cream for dessert, remember, you'd do equally well, if not better, smearing it on your face! Good luck... I hope you have as much fun with my beauty encyclopedia as I had in it's creation!

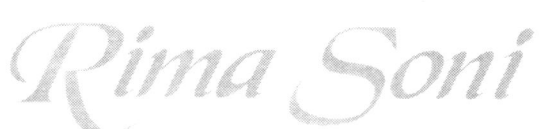

Food: The Goodness Within

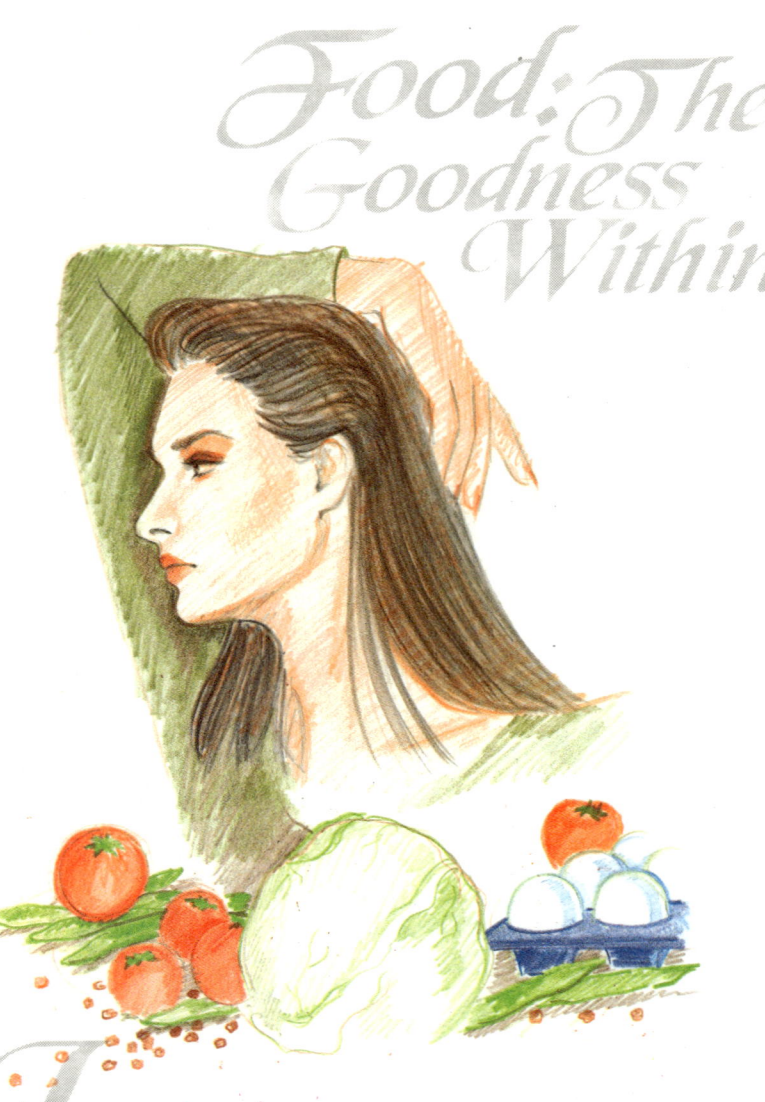

If you're concerned about your beauty, you're concerned about your health. Simply put, you are what you eat; you can't create something outside that isn't there within. Your metabolism converts food into energy, fueling you for work, play, growth, and the repair of body tissue. Metabolisms of course, vary: relaxed, easy going people are likely to put on weight at a faster rate than nervous hyperactives.

A balanced diet is essential to good health, and it's easy to commit yourself to eating well once you've mastered the basics of good, healthy eating. So, here goes —

FATS: You need fats -- present in all vegetables, oils, milk, cheese, meat, fish and poultry -- for good circulation and sleek, supple skin. Fat deposits protect the body from the cold and help preserve heat. Excessive fat, of course, leads to indigestion, obesity and heart disease. You need to monitor your fat intake -- eat more white meat and less red. Choose lean meat and remove all visible fat before cooking.

PROTEIN: Protein spurs growth and repairs and replaces body tissue. Present in meat, fish, eggs, milk and cheese, protein deficiencies cause dry skin and scalp, besides slowing the healing process. Protein needs peak during childhood, puberty and pregnancy. Vegetarians need to plan their diets carefully to include protein rich foods like soya beans, sprouts, cheese, milk, grains, mung beans, peas and kidney beans. Vegetables like peas and beans are good, low fat storehouses of protein. So are sprouted grains. In fact germinating seeds and grains enormously increase in nutritional value. Both the vitamin B and C content of mungbeans, lentils, soybean, fenugreek and beans increase by as much as 40 % during sprouting. Eggs, high in cholesterol, should be restricted to no more than 3 a week.

CARBOHYDRATES: Carbohydrate is converted into glucose, our chief source of energy. Foods like bread, flour and cereals provide your carbohydrate needs. A shortfall in this will be reflected in your energy level, so increase your consumption of wholemeal breads, nuts, honey, brown sugar and root vegetables.

INORGANIC SALTS: The body needs small amounts of iodine, calcium and iron for tissue building and repair. These inorganic salts are found in liver, watercress, fresh fish and green vegetables. A shortfall in your salt level can cause tooth decay, brittle nails, and a pallid skin.

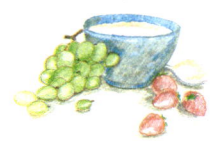

Breakfast

Oats, wheat or multi - grain porridge combined with milk or yogurt; or, a little cottage cheese followed by fruit. Infinitely better than fried eggs and sausages!

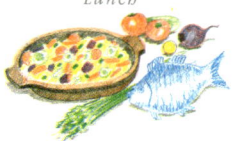

Lunch

Five different kinds of raw vegetables, tossed in a garlic, herb, olive oil and lemon dressing. Fish, chicken or nuts could be added to the salad. Wholegrain bread makes a great accompaniment.

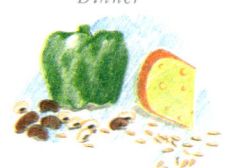

Dinner

Brown Rice or mixed beans and vegetables with a little cheese, flavored with onions, green peppers and herbs.

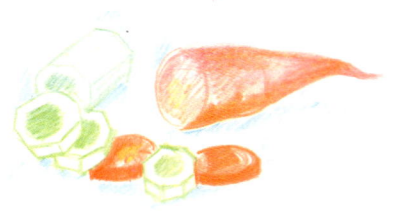

WATER: Your body is composed of 60 to 70 % fluids. Water is the original detoxicant, draining out toxics through perspiration and waste. It needs replacing. Fluids, of course, are important (ideally, consume 7-8 glasses of water daily); but small amounts of water are also present in the foods you consume. Less water causes blotchy, dull skin, and acne. But beware. Too much water can cause weight retention and a weight problem. Incidentally, a glass or two of water half an hour before meals aids digestion and restricts your appetite to amounts your body actually needs, curtailing the desire for excessive food.

VITAMINS: Chemical substances present in foods in minute quantities, vitamin deficiencies cause fatigue, lusterless hair, and a muddy complexion. Mountains of fresh fruit (perhaps a slice of fruit at every meal), fresh vegetables, honey, liver and yogurt will give you a vitamin enriched diet. Only take vitamin and mineral supplements if you don't feel fit despite healthy eating and a healthy lifestyle.

FIBRE: Fibre is vital, so make sure you get it in plenty. The indigestible carbohydrate concentrated in the peels and rinds of fruits and vegetables and in the outer layers of grains, fibre controls and regulates the process of food absorption, protecting against constipation and obesity. Fibre rich foods promote radiant, glossy skin and clear eyes.

How you eat your food is, of course, as important as what you eat. Fresh fruits and vegetables are better than cooked; steaming vegetables is preferable to boiling them. This ensures that important minerals (potassium in particular) aren't destroyed. Did you know that dicing or shredding vegetables with a knife depletes vitamin content? Chop or break vegetables, instead, into large chunks. This helps preserve vitamins.

Make it a point to replace refined flour with whole grain as, during the refining process, the outer husk -- or bran -- and the inner heart of the grain, rich in Vitamin B, protein and fibre are removed. What remains is just the starchy centre.

A marvelous cleansing technique is to adopt one day a week when you consume just mineral water, raw fruits and vegetables. This will release accumulated toxins, regenerate your metabolism and help shed unwanted flab. It will relax and revive you from the excesses of an unhealthy lifestyle. While fasting, skip cigarettes, alcohol, tea and coffee completely.

A rule of thumb to follow is : large breakfasts, medium lunches and small dinners. This ensures you are fueled for the whole day, with your protein and energy needs met in the morning. Alongside are some sample meals I follow. Tasty, nutritious, low-fat meals besides making you look and feel great, pep your energy levels enormously.

It's worth readjusting your diet. Believe me, eating foods right, and in the way nature intended will free you from an array of cosmetic products. You'll feel and look great, the way nature intended you to... so don't wait, start today!

KNOW YOUR VITAMINS

Vitamin A: Pineapple, mango, strawberries, vegetables, carrot, spinach, tomatoes, green leafy vegetables, milk, cream, cheese, butter, yogurt, chicken, liver, fish.
A deficiency of Vitamin A causes rough, scaly, skin, brittle nails and inflamed eyelids.

Vitamin B: Meat, liver, fish, poultry, lentils, cabbage, peas, beans, potatoes, coconut, milk, tomato, orange, bran, oatmeal, rye, almonds, nuts, peanuts. A shortfall in Vitamin B might cause acne, excessive weight, dandruff, falling hair, and a malfunctioning of the digestive system.

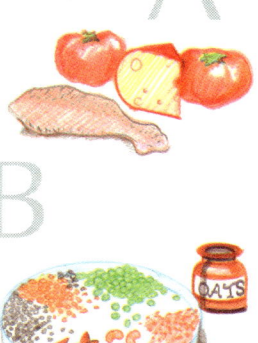

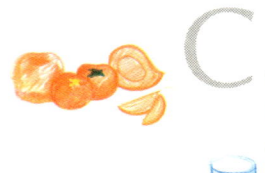

C

D

Vitamin C: Tomatoes, potaoes, carrot, turnips, cabbage, lemon, oranges, grapes, bananas, mangoes. Inadequate quantities of Vitamin C cause skin eruptions. If taken in sufficient amounts, this Vitamin cures health problems, helps reduce weight, and encourages healthy bones, gums and body tissue.

Vitamin D: Cod liver oil, milk, cheese, yogurt, eggs. A deficiency in Vitamin D can cause rickets, acne and brittle bones. Adequate supplys help prevent premature aging.

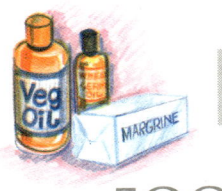

E

Vitamin E: Eggs, vegetable oils, peanut and wheatgerm oil, margerine. Besides helping cure hair problems, Vitamin E aids fertility and prevents premature ageing.

FOOD VALUES

If it's good enough to eat, its good enough to use in your beauty regime. Here are the nutritive and cosmetic values of certain food and non food items:

Avocado: A nutritious fruit, it contains vitamins, minerals and natural oils. Excellent for dry skins.

Almonds: I'd hate to underplay the value of this super nut! It improves skin, hair, nails. I use it in innumerable treatments and cleansers, to soften, nourish and cleanse.

Almond Oil: This rich oil nourishes the scalp and, when applied on dull, dry, skin, adds luster.

Apples: A natural skin toner and vitamin rich, apples shrink pores and tighten and tone skin. They also lighten skin. Being acidic, apples are astringent on oily skins.

Apricots: Rich in Vitamin A, apricots help refine coarse skin besides generally improving the skin's condition.

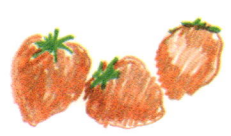
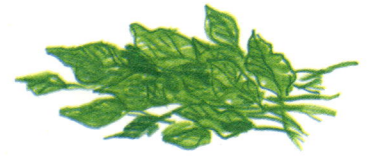

Bananas: Besides being nutritious to eat, bananas, used as masks are soothing and help prevent wrinkles. Mashed bananas with honey and cream besides tasting great, work wonders as masks for dry skin! For greasy, oily skins, blend them with a dash of orange juice.

Brewers Yeast: A rich source of Vitamin B and protein, Brewers Yeast cleanses, nourishes, tightens and activates circulation. Taken internally, it prevents dryness and acne. The tablets or powder help keep hair and skin glowing and shiny. Brewers Yeast helps stimulate blood to the skin, giving you added radiance and vitality.

Buttermilk: A fabulous cleanser, specially good for open pores. Also, a bleaching agent.

Bone Marrow: A nutritious hair treatment for falling hair, when warmed and applied on scalp. Works even better if left on overnight!

Camomile: Camomile has soothing and cleansing properties.

Carrots: Rich in Vitamin A, carrot pulp makes an effective mask. I use carrot oil in nourishing treatments and carrot juice in masks.

Coconut oil: Removes brown or black blemishes.

Coconut water, when dabbed on face and left on for 30 minutes, cures acne.

Cucumber: Rich in vitamins, cucumber is cooling, whitening and toning for the skin. Cucumber also refines the skin's pores.

Castor Oil: A rich oil, castor oil, if used daily on scanty lashes and eyebrows thickens them. Add some to your hair as a thickening agent.

Citrus fruits: are toning, astringent and antiseptic. Being acidic, they combat oiliness.

Cod Liver Oil: Rich in vitamin D, a capsule a day improves dry skin.

Corn Powder: I use this as a base, mixed with cream and honey, on dry skin. It is rich in Vitamin A.

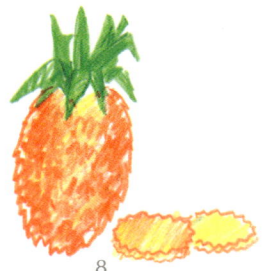

Dried Milk: Very nourishing for dry skin when mixed with yogurt and honey.

Eggs: The yolk, full of Lecithin and protein, is nourishing and enriching; the white - drying and tightening - tones, stimulates and keeps the skin feeling fresh for hours.

Glycerine: A humectant, which means that it attracts and holds moisture. A mixture of 100 ml glycerine and 1 tbsp lime juice, applied on dry skin every night helps keep skin soft and supple.

Garlic: Antiseptic properties. Taken daily, garlic helps reduce cholesterol thereby helping to guard against arteriosclerosis; It is also known to detoxify harmful substances. If you don't like taking it raw, buy garlic oil capsules. Also effective in treating pimple marks and boils.

Gelatin: A rich source of protein, gelatin strengthens nails and hair when eaten as a dessert or as a salad, mixed with raw vegetables, sprouts, cabbage, and cucumber.

Honey: Softens, moisturizes, nourishes, heals and cleanses skin.

Henna: An astringent herb with cooling properties. It is also a good hair dye and conditioner.

Lentils: Powdered lentils make great scrubs.

Lemon: Swimming in vitamin C, lemon juice is acidic, astringent, and bleaching. It is used in skin tonics.

Liver: Powerpacked with anti-stress vitamins and minerals like potassium sodium and magnesium.

Milk: Containing Vitamin D and Calcium, milk softens, nourishes and cleanses the skin. An effective cleanser, I use it in several masks to soften and cleanse.

Mint: A stimulating and refreshing herb. Used in skin tonics and masks.

Mayonnaise: This cosmetic cocktail boasts oil that lubricates, eggs that nourish, and vinegar to retain the acid mantle. Believe me, mayonnaise, being calorific, is best used for it's cosmetic rather than nutritive values.

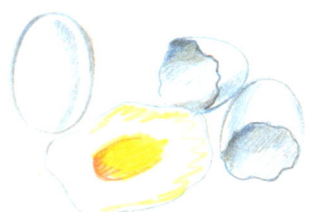

Olive oil: nourishing and lubricating.

Oats: An invigorating and softening skin scrub, oats contain Vitamin B and Calcium.

Onion : An antiseptic, onion is used in anti-wrinkle creams and is good for insommnia

Peaches: Refine coarse skin and improve skin condition.

Potato : Rich in Vitamin C, it helps cure pigmentation and uneven skin tones, apart from tightening pores.

Papaya: Rich in Vitamin A,B,C & D, papaya rejuvenates skin and improves the complexion.

Pineapple: Rich in Vitamin A, pineapple, mashed and applied on skin rejuvenates a dull complexion and removes dead cells.

Pumpkin Seeds: A complete protein, sprinkle on salads, fruits and vegetables.

Radish: Curbs formation of blackheads.

Salt: A great scrub and soothing in water for tired feet.

Strawberries: Great for their astringent properties, strawberries, with their Vitamin A content, lighten and even skin tone. Especially good for oily skins, it's enzymes help to tone a tired oily skin reducing the oils and refining the pores. Strawberries also fade tans.

Sugar: An abrasive face scrub, great for cleansing and toning skin.

Sprouted grains: A powerhouse of good 'live food' nourishment. An excellent source of protein, mineral, complex carbohydrate, vitamins and small quantities of essential fatty acids.

Tomatoes: Rich in vitamins, tomatoes are natural skin softeners. They reduce oiliness, shrink pores, lighten skin and tone complexion.

Tea: Soothes tired eyes and conditions hair. Use cool tea bags to cool and freshen eyes.

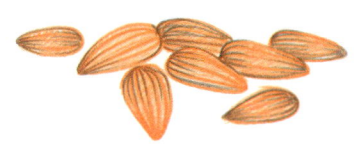

Vinegar: The skin has an acid mantle, and vinegar, being acidic, restores this. Used as a final hair rinse, it conditions and improves dry, itchy scalp. A final vinegar rinse after a shower helps to keep skin smooth and conditioned. Vinegar balances the PH of skin.

Watermelon: Helps to refine coarse skin. As a toner and a lightener, it improves skin condition.

Witch hazel: Basically an astringent, witch hazel is used to close pores. Eye pads soaked in cool water and witch hazel is said to soothe tired eyes.

Yeast: Bakers yeast is rich in Vitamin B complex. It makes an excellent face mask.

Yogurt: Rich in protein, calcium, and vitamins, yogurt is used in facial masks for oily and dull skins. This dairy product contains bacteria which keep the intestines clean and calcium to clear blemished skin and calm troubled nerves. Yogurt makes an excellent hair conditioner.

For masks using the ingredients listed above, see section on treatments. Treatments using these and other ingredients will be listed in the relevant chapters. For instance, the treatment for chapped and coarse knees will be included in the chapter on Legs.

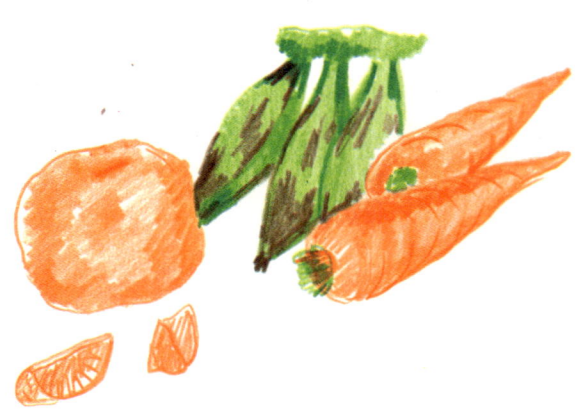

The Enemy Within... Your Food

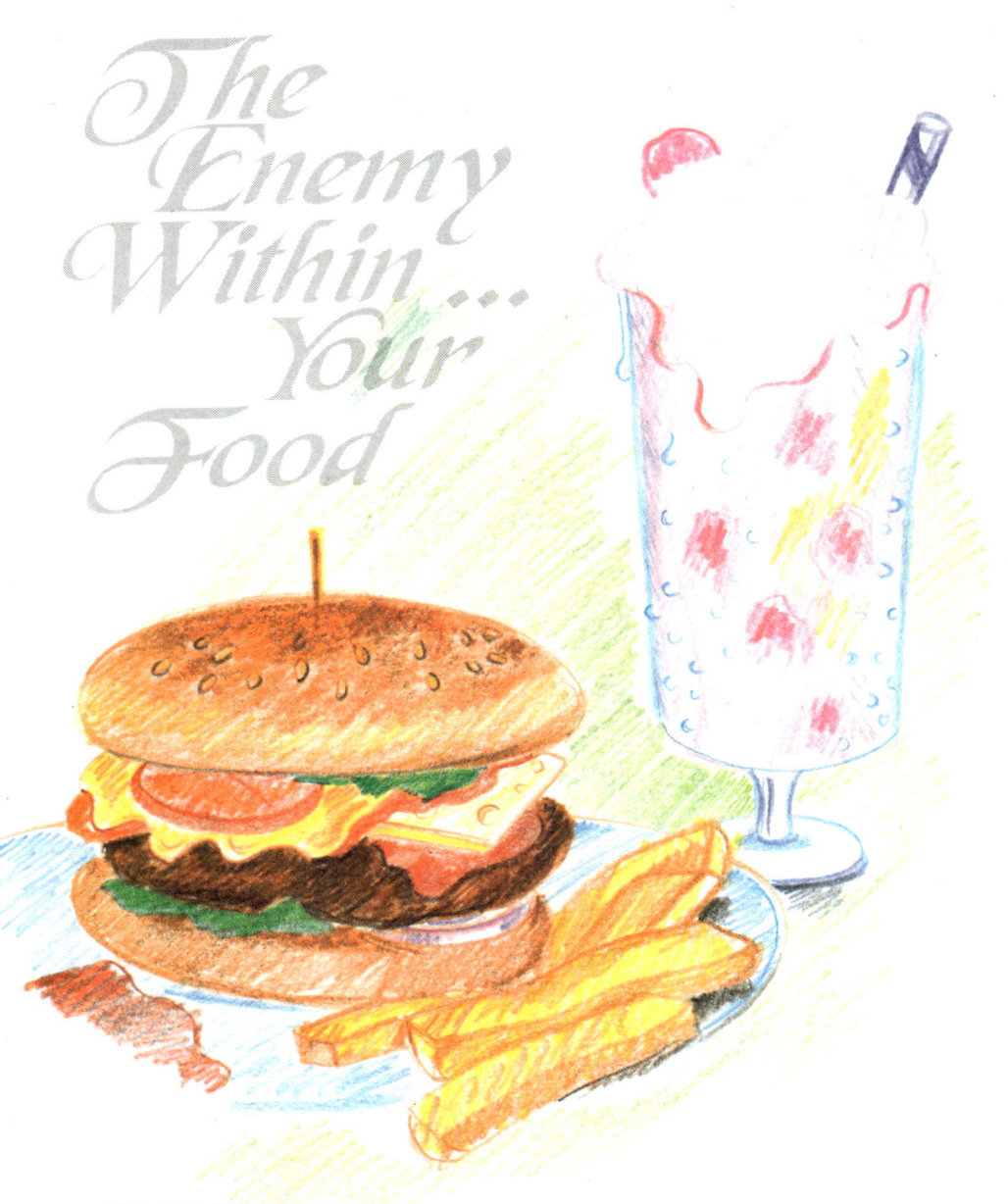

We'd all love radiant, glowing looks, and infinite energy that propels us to achieve the impossible. To achieve this, we'd probably need to readjust our lifestyle and take a hard look at ourselves and what we eat.

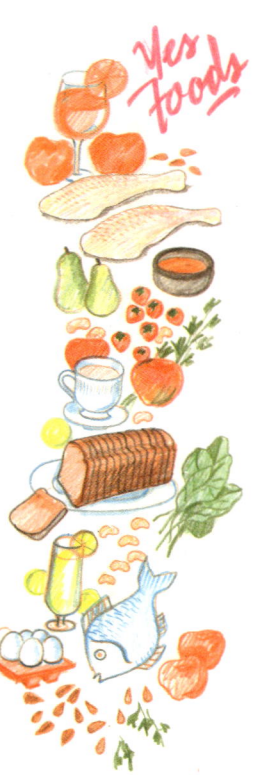

The food you eat can enhance or sully the way you look, not unlike your environment. Stay away from your favorite sunrisers, both coffee and tea, as, taken with milk and sugar, they are calorific; taken excessively, they clog pores and prevent toxins from being eliminated from the body. Caffeine, nutritionally a zero, may give you a chemically induced, temporary 'high'. But you'd do well instead (and get a natural boost) by starting your mornings with a cup of herbal tea.

If you want to preserve your good looks and joie de vivre, do avoid the whole battery of refined and processed products that fill supermarkets today with their glitzy packaging and appeal. Heading the list is refined sugar. Since its main nutrients and the enzymes necessary for its utilisation are processed out, sugar. has no value. On the contrary, it can cause acne, poor circulation and obesity. Instead, add brown sugar or honey to your diet. Both help purify blood and cleanse the body of toxins. And of course -- nothing can touch the nutritional goodness of fruit sugars present in raw fruit. Fruit binges are entirely acceptable... literally, even too much is not enough! Avoid chocolates too, as, being heating, they cause clogged pores.

Other 'whole' foods rich in Vitamins B, E and other vital nutrients are whole grains. Substitute wholewheat bread for white, brown rice for refined, and other fibre-rich refined cereals for refined, packaged ones. Foods should be eaten the way they were meant to be, with nothing added or taken away. Unrefined foods prevent skin disorders, improve digestion, help control blemishes and maintain the level of collagen in the body.

Add bran to your diet as it helps balance skin condition as well as aid digestion.

Reduce your salt intake. especially if you tend towards puffiness around the eyes and a bloating feeling around your menstrual cycle. Even if you don't, your salt intake should be minimal as most foods in their natural form contain salt.

Smoking is outlawed. Possibly, your greatest enemy, I can't overstate it's evils. Smoking constricts blood vessels, dehydrates the skin and causes an ugly network of lines to appear around the lips and eyes. Smoking also causes premature aging by stressing the pancreas and adrenals. After your lungs, the worst hit is your skin: smoking depletes the supply of Vitamin C, producing acid smoke which pollutes the skin's surface.

Spicy foods, too, are taboo. Beware of them; research studies today indicate that a spicy diet can actually become a physical addiction, your body begins to crave it! Excessive spice can dilate blood vessels and rupture capillaries under the skin, causing an ugly network of lines to appear. Spicy foods can also cause an unnatural flush color as well as eruptions on the skins surface. Far from improving digestion, spices actively inhibit the draining out of toxins from your body. Conventional wisdom dictates you don't read a book by it's cover. I, in fact, believe you do. Simply put, you are what you eat. The environment you create within you is reflected in your eyes, your skin, your smile. So remember, You're in control. Make the right choices. Now, is not too late!

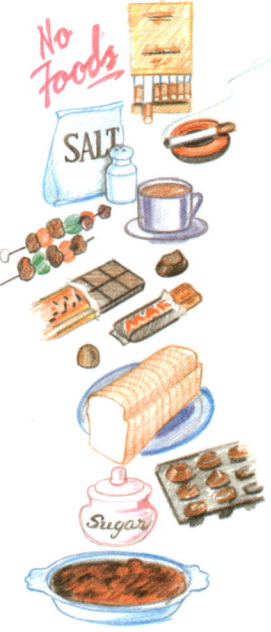

Softer, Smoother Skin

We've all been through phases when everyone's skin seems more spotless, clear, and smooth than ours. They've probably worked at it. For, maintaining a radiant complexion isn't easy, but the rewards are worth it. Skin should never be neglected as the epidermis layer will deteriorate. Irregular cleansing, for instance, will cause a buildup of dead cells, ruining the skins condition.

Never make lame excuses."I'm too busy" just isn't good enough. You owe it to yourself to look good. So, no matter what time you return home in the evening, your skin must be thoroughly cleansed, as no amount of make-up and camouflage will hide your skin's real condition.

For that healthy glow, diet is important. Avoid junk foods, carbonated drinks, chocolates, and heavy moghlai dishes, concentrating instead on cottage cheese, whole meal breads, green leafy vegetable, fresh fruits, fresh juices and plenty of water. Introduce a skin care regimen to your daily routine, that besides nourishing foods, includes rest, fresh air and exercise. Cleansing, toning, moisturising and a facial mask once a week will help you achieve your goal - skin that glows with inner radiance and vitality. Moisturise your skin every night, but - dab carefully under the eyes, as night creams, massaged in the wrong direction can cause deeper lines. If the skin around your neck is sagging or loose, concentrate your massage here.

Make sure your skin is always clear of blackheads and white heads. It is always advisable to use a scrub in the case of blackheads. Facial masks straight from your kitchen or back garden are quick, low cost pick-me-ups during the hot summer months, giving you a cool tingling feeling. Use seasonal fruit: papaya, strawberry, banana or pineapple. Pulp it and spread it. A later chapter on facials, masks and treatments will give you a whole range of fruity masks.

Wrinkles have many causes, including sun, dehydration, and sudden weight loss. Always wear goggles and moisturise your skin before stepping out as squinting causes ugly lines around the eyes and on the forehead. Water, of course, is a great wrinkle preventer as it flushes out toxins from your body and reduces dehydration.

The aging process, too, affects the skin's normal functioning causing lines and making it dull and lifeless. This of course, needn't be. Though the aging process cannot be stopped, it can be stemmed. Use an exfoliating mask once a week to remove dead skin cells and dry patches.

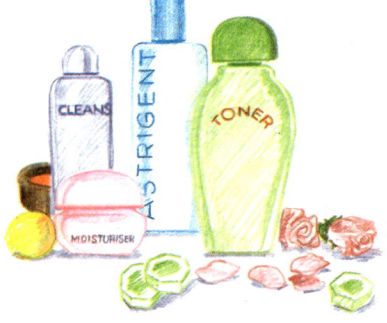

For Oily Skins

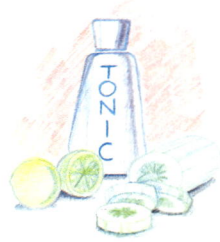

Make a skin tonic by adding a few drops of lime juice to a spoonful of cucumber juice. This combined mixture improves a dull and greasy complexion.

For Normal Skin

Oat paste works as an excellent scrub. You may also foment your face with a solution of 1/2 cup boiling water and 1/2 tsp baking soda. Great for loosening blackheads, and pressing them out.

Mix one tsp oats, one tsp almond powder and rosewater to make a paste. Then add one tsp honey. Mix well and leave on skin for 15 minutes. Rinse off with cold water. Pat on moisturiser.

For mature skins

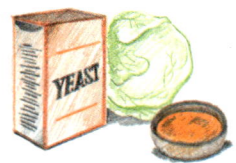

Dissolve 1 tsp. yeast in one tsp cabbage juice. Mix with one tsp. honey. Smooth the mask on laughter lines and crows feet, avoiding the eye area, then extend to your face and neck. Leave on for 15 minutes. Remove gently with a damp napkin. This mask helps smooth lines and close pores.

This will give your skin a sheen. Wear a natural mask once a week. It closes pores and improves circulation.

Ten minutes of daily exercise will improve blood circulation, nourishing your skin further. And please don't diet excessively. A little (but just a little) fat deposit under the skin holds and supports it, making it appear smoother. When I need to lose weight I exercise, rather than diet and I advise you to do the same. Exercise boosts your metabolism which automatically burns up extra calories.

Smoking dehydrates your skin, creating furrows above the top lip. Each cigarette depletes you of as much as 25mg. of vitamin C, a vitamin important to the production of collagen. This is why smoking is said to cause premature aging, negating your good looks.

A professional massage has to be professionally executed, so, never try massaging your face at home. A monthly visit to a beautician helps. Her scientific and professional strokes will invigorate your skin. Besides this, she'll be able to concentrate on problem areas. Finally, your skin will reflect your mental state as nothing else will. Happiness, the best cosmetic, is vital for your looks. Remember, frowning tenses 50 facial muscles and laughing relaxes 13! Whenever you feel tense withdraw to a quiet corner of the house. Inhale deeply, 10 to 15 times, and think positive thoughts. You'll feel better instantly!

Your face speaks for you, more than words. Boredom, ill temper, and irritation all get inscribed on your face. In time they become indelible. Serenity, humour, kindness and contentment lend the face an inner beauty and charm. Your temperament begins to affect the way you look from your 20s. By the time you're 50, your face owes more to you than to nature. Besides a happy breezy temperament, exaggerated facial expressions encourage line formation and wrinkles that a little self awareness can avoid.

A skin regime should be selected according to skin type. Perform this small experiment first: wash your face before retiring. Do not apply anything; leave your skin clean. In the morning, check your skin by wiping with a dry tissue.

If the tissue has oil on it you have an oily skin. If the oil is only on a 'T' shape this indicates your forehead, nose and chin are oily. This is a combination skin. If there is no oil you may either have a normal or a dry skin. A dry skin feels stretched after a soap wash whereas a normal skin is smooth. Let's go step by step through the different skin types and treatments:-

Normal skin: Normal skin looks smooth, supple and unblemished with no enlarged pores. The only time it may pimple is during menstruation when hormonal changes cause the sebaceous glands to overactivate. Normal skin requires a cleansing cream, tonic and moisturiser. A mask every ten days is freshening. Use rose water as a skin tonic. Almond powder, milk powder and honey works wonders as a complete face pack - so all a person with normal skin needs to carry is ground almonds, milk powder, rose water and honey!

If you have a combination skin, use a cleansing lotion for the 'T' and a cleansing cream for the cheeks. Then tone your skin with astringent on the T and tonic on the cheeks. A facial pack once every 10 days is beneficial.

Mature skin: This skin requires daily attention: Pamper it with cleansing creams, tonics, rich moisturisers and night creams. A light, firming face mask like the one delineated in the column is very beneficial.

Dry skin: A dry skin needs cleanser, tonic and a mask. The cleanser should be of whole milk, so carry whole milk powder and olive oil. First mix the whole milk to make liquid and add 1/2 tsp. olive oil. Use this as your cleanser, rosewater as a tonic and the facial mask I've described in the treatment column to tone.

Oily skin: Prone to acne and clogged pores, oily skin needs cleansing at least three times a day. The treatments described work wonders on this skin type!

Masks are essential for all skin types as they have myriad benefits: they nourish, cleanse, tighten, smooth, tone and freshen the skin. But masks work best when both body and mind are relaxed. 20 minutes is all your skin demands from you.

For dry skins

1 tsp cornflour,
1 tsp whole milk made
into a paste with
and 1 tsp. honey
is a wonderful
face mask for dry skin.

For Oily skin

Skimmed milk powder
with 2 drops of
concentrated lime juice
is a thorough cleanser.
Rose water with Oat powder,
honey and lemon juice,
is also effective.

An oily skin also
requires a gritty skin scrub.
Nothing could be simpler
than a little sugar
with a dash of lemon
juice before your mask.

*A great
beauty mask*

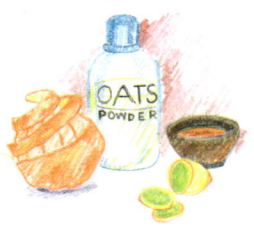

Mix 1 tsp
orange peel powder,
1 tblsp. oats powder,
1 tsp. honey and
3 drops lemon juice
in rose water.
Make this into a thick
paste and apply on face.

Bleaches

For children, use a fine paste of almonds, milk and a pinch of turmeric powder on the wet body instead of soap. Gently scrub the body with the paste. A few drops of lemon juice can be added for school going children.

A cool summer bleach can be prepared from mashed strawberries mixed with butter milk. Proportion: four strawberries to one tblsp. buttermilk.

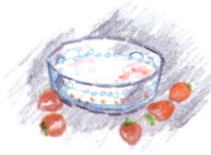

To wear off tan and soothe sunburn, rub tanned areas with yogurt, buttermilk, cucumber or tomato slices.

Don't let your genes have the final say, as believe me, you can transform the colour and tone of your skin. The skin constantly regenerates itself. Your complexion's capacity for change is enormous -- you just need to help it reach it's potential.

AVOID SUN BURN

Exposure to the sun's rays can permanently damage your skin by destroying the collagen layers that support it, resulting in wrinkling. The secret of Joan Collins' youthful looks is that she avoids the sun.

Small children require sunlight for vitamin D. But even so, I recommend you under rather than over-expose as too much sun damages and depletes the skin over a period of time. It causes premature aging, crows feet and deep lines on the forehead. It lowers the absorption of vitamin B, which helps improve skin, complexion and hair. It also overbleaches hair, destroying it's texture besides darkening and deepening pigmentation and freckles.

Sensitive skin can burn and peel with excessive exposure to the sun. It's advisable, always, to cover your body with a sunscreen. Hats, scarves and large glasses that protect the sides of the eyes are essential to keep crows feet at bay. Remember, too, that the sun can dehydrate the skin making it thick and leathery. Natural bleaching packs like those that combine yogurt, oats and powdered almonds work wonders. If you're suffering from sun burn or blisters, cucumber slices gently rubbed will soothe the affected areas. To be really effective, all sunburn treatments should be executed for at least half an hour.

STRETCH MARKS

Stretch marks aren't just caused by childbirth - they can follow weight loss, puberty, and at times, are hereditary.

The areas generally affected are the stomach, hips, thighs, bust and back of the arms. Stretch marks are long, thin, white lines on the skin surface. When the skin stretches - due to weight gain or other factors, it's dermal layer is damaged, and the skin breaks beneath the surface, leaving lines.

Supple skin, made so by lubricating the entire body with warm olive oil; especially on the stomach and breasts during weight loss stages, will help prevent stretch marks. This should be done after a bath, when the body is still wet. The body, then, should be gently towelled. Repeat this twice weekly.

People with taut and dry skin are more likely to be victims of stretch marks. Zinc gives elasticity and collagen to the skin, besides encouraging cell growth. Foods rich in zinc are seafoods, like oysters and herrings. Take zinc tablets if the skin is dry and prone to stretch marks. However if you're expecting, check with you doctor if it's contraindicated during pregnancy.

Stretch Marks

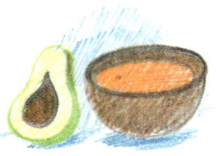

Take an avocado and make it into a pulp. Mix one tsp. of honey and spread the paste over dry areas and those prone to stretch marks. Relax in the tub for 30 minutes and rinse off with lukewarm water. Follow this with the olive oil treatment.

NO SWEAT OVER PERSPIRATION

Perspiration enables the body to rid itself of toxins. Everyone perspires and if you perspire a lot, there's no need to feel ashamed. After all, we have over two million sweat glands distributed all over the body! Perspiration is the body's natural cooling system. Occasionally, we might perspire due to pungent foods, hot drinks like tea or coffee, physical fatigue, fear, excitement, temperature or, of course, because of the type of fabrics we wear.

There are two types of sweat glands - the eccrine glands, which are clear, salty and odorless and the apocrine glands, found mainly under the arms and between the legs. Children below nine years do not have apocrine glands. The main reason for odour in sweat is due to bacteria on the skin in body areas where moisture cannot evaporate easily. Pungent foods also cause odorous sweat. To avoid perspiration always deodorize your body, allowing it to dry on the skin before wearing clothes.

A natural treatment to keep body odour at bay is a solution of lemon rind, rose petals and mint leaves. Boil and leave overnight. In the morning, dip a dry napkin in the solution and dab over the entire body, especially, your underarms, neck, feet and hands. Let it dry. Now, sprinkle some talc if you wish. This homemade lotion can be prepared every third day. Besides reducing body odour, it also reduces perspiration.

Deodorant

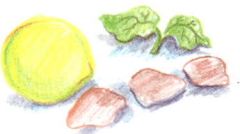

Mint, lemon rind and rose petal solution

WATER POWER

Your skin holds moisture. It stands to reason, then, that water makes it soft and supple. When it loses moisture, it becomes dry and tight. I cannot underestimate the importance of water for healthy skin. Cold water stimulates the skin, shocking it into a nice pink glow. Hot water baths relax and soothe the body lessening fatigue and pain. Hot baths are also soporific, (so enjoy them before a bath); and healthy as they induce perspiration which helps eliminate bacteria. But caution -- hot baths, if overdone, deplete your body of energy and tone. On the other hand, to increase your energy levels, vitality and disease resistance, luxuriate in any one of the cold or treatment baths I've described.

Water has the remarkably magical property of altering the body state. The addition of natural products help. Some products for instance, hasten perspiration to stimulate the release of stored toxins within the body.

An oats bath is excellent for skin ailments. It soothes, softens, overcomes itchiness, relieves sunburn, and gets rid of dead cells, leaving the body smooth and silky. A vinegar bath is an excellent cosmetic for skin. One cup of vinegar dissolved in water conditions your skin, restoring the body's natural acid covering. Salt baths rejuvenate if you've had a string of late nights. Just rub coarse salt onto your back and entire body carefully avoiding your face. Or, add three teaspoons of salt in your bath water. This will help relax and refresh you.

For skin ailments

Wrap a cup of oats in muslin. Drop it into your bath water. While in the bath, scrub the soaked muslin gently over skin. Relax with the muslin immersed in water for 15 minutes. Now take a cool shower.

To smoothen wrinkles

Wrap some ice cubes in muslin and place in bowl. Cream or oil your face. As the ice melts, splash your face with icy water several times; moving from your cheeks, to your forehead, eyes and throat. Rubber gloves will prevent your hands getting numb. Dab skin with a napkin and moisturise.

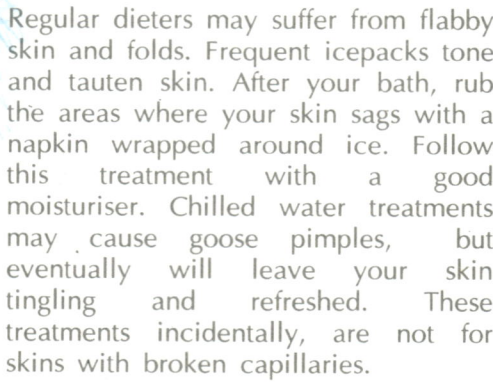

Regular dieters may suffer from flabby skin and folds. Frequent icepacks tone and tauten skin. After your bath, rub the areas where your skin sags with a napkin wrapped around ice. Follow this treatment with a good moisturiser. Chilled water treatments may cause goose pimples, but eventually will leave your skin tingling and refreshed. These treatments incidentally, are not for skins with broken capillaries.

ORANGE PEEL SKIN

Concentrated fat in certain parts of the body which makes the skin look like orange peel is called Cellulite.

Caused by sluggish metabolism, due mainly to a poor diet, inadequate water and exercise, cellulite occurs more frequently in women than men. It may be hereditary, or caused during puberty, pregnancy or menopause. And of course, if you're overweight, you're most likely to get it than if you're not. The most common areas for cellulite formation are the hips, thighs, buttocks and knees.

High protein, green leafy vegetables, tomatoes and radish, are great for orange peel skin.

Cut carbohydrates and sugar from your diet and replace them with high protein meats, green leafy vegetables, plenty of cucumber (with the skin), tomatoes, radish, cabbage, carrots, spinach and fresh fruits like strawberries, pineapples, grapefruits and apples. Eat unsalted nuts and cheese. In fact, try and reduce your salt intake.

Water, especially mineral, helps. Replace tea with herbal teas and avoid coffee and water between meals. Coffee aggravates cellulite. Special gels and soaps are available for cellulite problems. Massage the lumpy areas with gloves with leather spikes available at the pharmacy. Make sure you massage upwards, clockwise or anti-clockwise.

When visiting health clubs -- particularly those which have a jet massage fitted - make sure you target it to cellulite areas. Vibrator belts and rollers also help in keeping cellulite at bay. Be particularly gentle in your treatment, though, if you have varicose veins.

Exercise plays a vital role in Cellulite control. Walking, swimming and cycling in the air are helpful. There are other special exercises like the shoulder stand that help shift cellulite which can be learned from trained practitioners or Yoga experts.

Those Tumultuous Teens

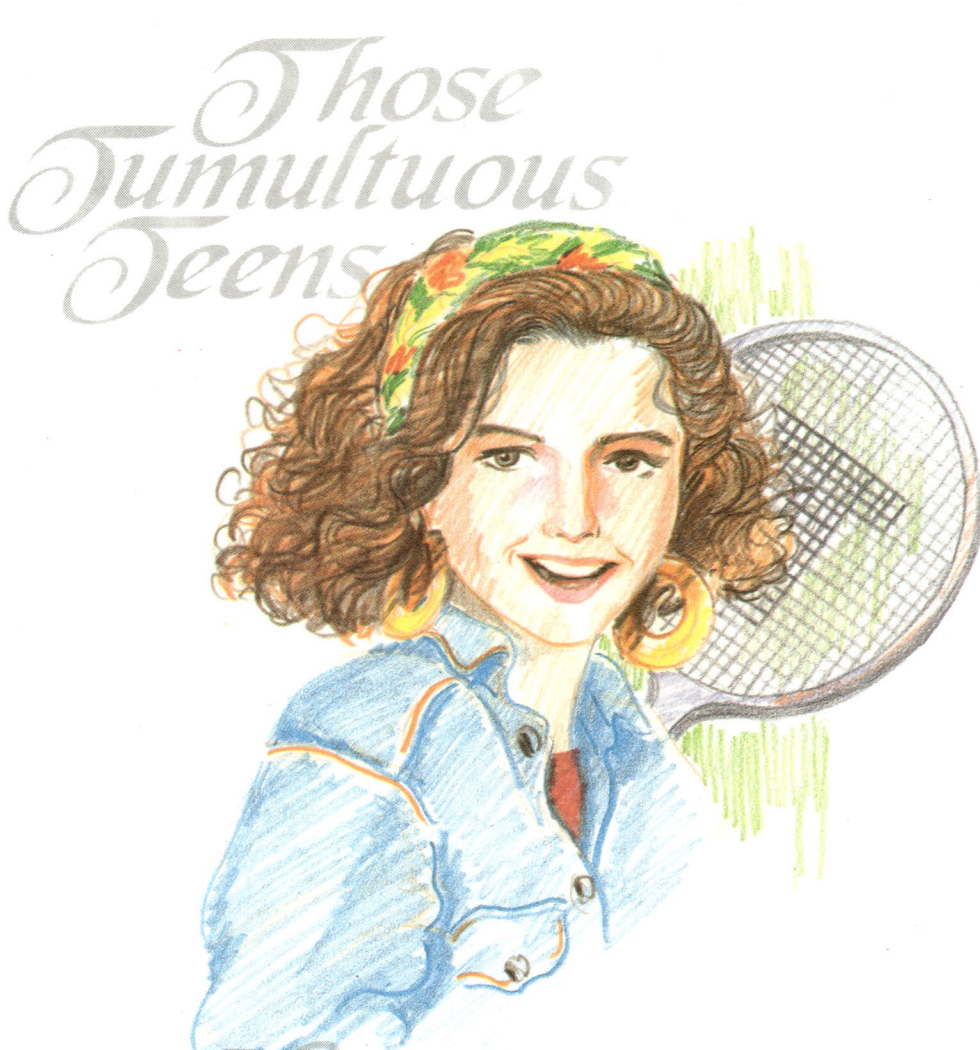

Your teens are a time for revelry; for being your busiest, and hopefully, looking your best. You're probably looking and feeling sensational, and you'll look the same no matter which grooming rule you make and break. However, I'd recommend that every teenager start today, laying the foundation for a great looking future ! Start at 13, start with a little bit of self awareness; as your particular set of problems and lifestyle will require a separate beauty regime.

TOWARDS RADIANT SKIN

Your skin is possibly oily, as oil secretions during your teen years tend to peak due to hormonal changes. This might lead it to appear grimy, especially during summer, as the oil secreted attracts dust and dirt. If you suffer from an oily skin it is absolutely essential that you cleanse your skin at least two to three times a day. Soap isn't adequate; you need to use a cleanser to tackle the grime.

Once cleansed, it has to be wiped off with damp cotton till the skin is squeaky clean. Now, close your pores by splashing chilled water in which you've squeezed 1/2 a lemon. This skin tonic reduces oil, closes pores and makes your skin tingle! Really, that's all you need! You can carry your cleanser, concentrated lemon juice and cotton in your handbag to help you look fresh and radiant all day.

As a natural cleanser skimmed milk is great. It also helps to remove makeup completely. Tomatoes and potatoes too, act as skin cleansers. Just rub them on the skin to remove dead skin and excessive oils.

But first, let's do a quick run-through of your skin: the skin is composed of the epidermis or outer layer, which consists of keratin cells that are constantly sloughed off and replaced. Within the epidermis are specialised cells called Melanocytes. They produce melanin i.e. the pigmentation which gives you colour.

The collagen containing dermis, which gives elasticity contains tiny blood vessels that nourish the nails, hair and skin. Blood capillaries, sweat glands and hair roots are also situated here. The dermal layer determines the shape or contour of the body and face. The sebaceous glands are the oil glands in the dermal layer. Sebum is a semi-liquid consisting of oil mixed with water and waste matters. With normal stimulation, sebum oozes out in slight amounts. If the circulation is unbalanced or the gland activity, retarded, the sebum hardens and plugs the pores, forming blackheads.

Skins react magically to nurturing and the environment.

Oily Skin

Mix a tbsp. of camomile with 2 tbsp. hot water and leave for 10 minutes. Strain. Mix the camomile liquid with oats to make a paste and add 1/2 tsp. honey.

Use a tomato toner.

Dab tomato juice on your skin with cotton wool. The acid content of tomato helps clean pores and discourage blackheads.

Face Scrub

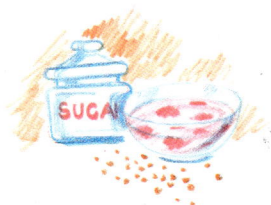

Take a tsp. of sugar and mix it with one tsp. of oats. Add a little water to make a paste. Gently scrub your face, concentrating on the nose, chin and cheeks. Follow this with a dab of rose water and a touch of moisturiser.

Both can cause it's functioning and texture, tone and colour to improve or deteriorate. An improper diet and insufficient water, too, will take a toll on our skin. There are, of course, other factors beyond our control, that need countering. These include wind, cold, heat, and air pollution.

To stay young and healthy, normal skin requires a regular routine of cleansing, stimulation and protection with a milk cleanser and lemon and water, to retain it's intrinsic radiance.

Oily skin, often the result of hot humid weather and improper skin care can cause acne, open pores and blackheads. It is prone to infection as oil trapped at the base of the pore shafts creates an environment in which germs thrive. Usually, adolescents tend towards oily skins as, during this time, the sebaceous glands secrete sebum to supply the skin's surface with a protective grease. This can cause infection, open pores and germs to enter freely. Whiteheads and blackheads, too, tend to proliferate. Cleanse your skin at least twice a day - mornings and nights. If you have oily skin, pimples and acne don't necessarily follow. People with healthy eating habits who exercise regularly and follow a religious skin care routine usually have oily skin with no blemishes.

Black heads or comedones can be black, brown or white. They are dried sebaceous secretions, usually mixed with keratin and the debris of cells that line skin pores. Forerunners of acne, they mainly occur during adolescence when the sebaceous glands are overactive. Treat blackheads with a strict cleansing routine. Never pick them without steaming your face. Steaming will help soften pores so you can remove them easily. Avoid using milk cleansers on this skin type. If you do, remove with damp cotton wool and dab on astringent - as this helps tone the skin and improve circulation. It gives a tingling freshness to an otherwise sluggish complexion.

Stay away from fried foods, soft drinks and white sugar. Substitute this with fresh fruits, vegetables, juices, and fish. Add brewers yeast to your daily diet -as this helps normalise oily skin condition.

Model Looks

If you've been looking at Cosmopolitan and Vogue, enviously wondering how models look the way they do, I have some tips passed on to me by some model friends for you:
When their skin looks dreary, they whip up a skin snack, really, a kind of mayonnaise using egg white, undersaturated oil, apple cider vinegar, water and lecithin (which isn't cheating) .Then, when they're sure the doorbell won't ring, they cover their skin with this mixture (never forgetting the neck), and the skin seems to drink it up. After only a few moments .the skin's texture and elasticity improve.

Milk, an emulsion of 3.8 % butterfat and water, stabilised by about 3% in protein, is cosmetically powerful, as the big boys in the cosmetic business know.

And to wrap up, dab translucent powder before your makeup to prevent the oiliness from shining through.

The sun, heat, cold and wind can evaporate the skins water, causing dryness. Cold weather is uncomfortable for a person with dry skin as it de-activates the skin's oil secretions, causing the skin to peel. Dry skin comes with another package of problems: your pores, if blocked, will cause infection to be trapped under the skin's surface, causing spots. Dry skin is sometimes caused by neglecting your diet and skin care routine. Insufficient water draws out the reserves from the skin in the form of perspiration and water. Dry skins require milk cleansers, toners and nourishing night creams.

The following ground rules apply to all skin types:

Drink at least two bottles of water every day. Keep them in your room to ensure you don't forget. Water is vital for all skin problems: in dry skin cases it provides moisture and in oily skins it drains out toxins.

Check your bowel movements. If you're constipated, use natural foods to cure the problem rather than pills. Have foods like papaya, milk with honey or All-bran with milk.

The epidermis layer constantly flakes off, and is replaced by cells from the layer below. Apply friction, like an oats-sugar rub every fourth day to remove flaked cells ... and watch that skin glow!.

Cleanse skin thoroughly nights and mornings. Tone by splashing the skin with cold water or patting with skin tonic. Skin tonic is an instant vitaliser. Always have on a light moisturiser. Remember too, to sleep enough. Exercise and outdoor activity (see the chapter on exercise) also stimulates blood circulation and tones the body.

They also zip up their circulation with cider vinegar, using one part vinegar to eight parts water, with a dash of fresh grapefruit juice. The cider vinegar helps the skin retain it's natural moisture content, while the grapefruit juice - lemon and watermelon would do as well - containing between 5 to 8 % citric acid, helps keep the balance This recipe, my model informants tell me, reduces the chance of blemishes.

AN IDEAL DIET

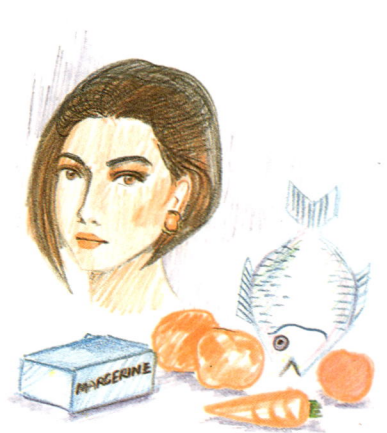

Ensure you get an adequate supply of Vitamin - A.

As a teenager you're under constant academic and physical pressure. Healthy food is directly linked to how you look and feel.

Certainly don't ban hamburgers, Kentucky fried chickens, icecreams and colas but counter their effect with heaps of nutritional foods.

Never skip meals. If you don't have time to eat breakfast, try my complete "Beauty drink" - a glass of juice which is a combination of spinach, parsley and oranges liquidised and sieved. Rich in iron and vitamin 'C', it's great for a clear complexions.

Or try the other banana based complete food drink I've concocted. Blend a banana with a tablespoon of brewers yeast powder and a glass of milk. I love this concoction as it gives me instant energy besides providing me with calcium, iron and B complex.

By eating well, you're not just indulging your skin, you're looking after every part of your body. Give your hair as much importance as your skin, in fact, pamper your hair. As hair is made up of protein, a protein diet works wonders! If you're going through a tense or unwell period, increase your protein intake. Make sure your diet includes milk, cheese, eggs, fruit and salads.

Vitamin B complex is essential for hair. Take six tablets of brewers yeast tablets for dull or falling hair. Better still, mix one teaspoon brewers yeast in your glass of juice. Your health and vitality are finally reflected in your eyes. Ensure you get plenty of Vitamin A, present in carrots, oranges, apricots, margarine, butter, sardines, salmon, tuna, and herrings. For sparkling, larger than life eyes, take a cod-liver oil capsule daily.

COPING WITH ACNE

I'm devoting an entire section to acne; as this teenage grouse can mar your adolescent years! Caused due to hormonal changes and an oversecretion of sebacoues glands, Vulgaris, the most common kind of acne, is easy to cure. All it takes is plenty of water to rid the system of toxins. Also, steer clear of starchy foods, coffee, cocoa and sweets as they cause sluggish circulation.

Do not take any medication or apply ointments without a doctor's recommendation. Picking at the acne only worsens the condition and causes blemishes. Stress and worry don't help, so soothe your nerves with a camomile drink. You might have noticed, for instance, that just before exams, your acne might alarmingly multiply!

Cleansing the skin at least thrice daily helps infections and a daily facial mask improves severe skin conditions. If, after trying some home grown treatments and cures straight from the kitchen, you find your skin condition hasn't improved, consult a doctor.

I've noticed that teenagers desperately resort to strong treatments to clear acne. I recommend you take it easy and concentrate on improving your diet. Drink at least 10 glasses of water a day and exercise to keep that circulation on a high! Start on a skin regime that keeps your skin immaculate always and make sure your digestive system is working just so. If it isn't, clean your system once a month with natural laxatives. You might even fast one day in a month. Eat just papaya or pineapple - these fruits are nutritive and help flush toxins from your body and cleanse your complexion.

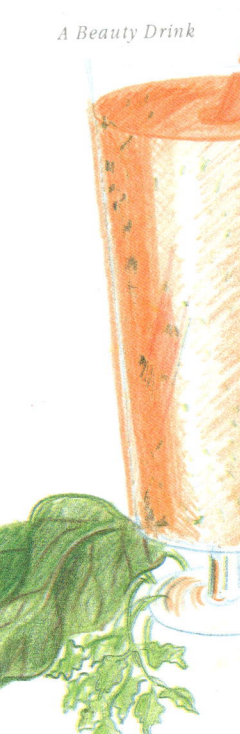

A Beauty Drink

The second type of acne is acne frontalis This has yellowish scales and appears usually on the forehead and temples and around the hairline. Check with your dermatologist for treatment.

The third kind of acne, acne rosacea, normally affects women over thirty. Caused by scurf or indigestion, it's main characteristics are red cheeks, chin and nose.

It's important to relax, take walks in the fresh air and avoid getting emotionally upset as the redness increases with stress. Give up starchy foods, hot tea and coffee and avoid climatic extremes.

I advise every young girl, wholeheartedly, to incorporate natural cleansers, tonics and masks in her skin care routine. Of course, there's a time factor involved in using pure foods and potions handed down from our grandmothers. Off the shelf products might work quicker... but you can feel the difference for yourself !

ARMS AND LEGS

Do you dream of unimaginably long, smooth, legs and arms? Don't ever write this off as a distant dream; all you require is a little exercise to overcome flabby arms and legs. To begin with, rotate your arms clockwise and anti-clockwise at least 10 times every day.

Legs, too, can be made more shapely and smooth, and the time to start is now, during your teen years. Stand straight, resting your arms on the chair back rest. Swing the right leg as high as possible and bring back to position without touching the ground. Do this continuously, 10 times. Now work on the other leg. This reduces pudginess in your thigh area, giving you a long legged look.

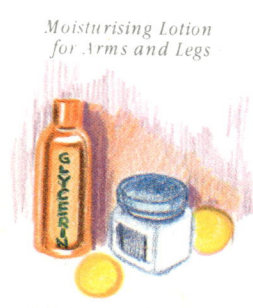

Moisturising Lotion for Arms and Legs

6 tbsps. petroleum jelly, 2 tbsp glycerine, 1\2 tsp. of lemon juice. Mix well and apply all over your arms and legs. Dab this on your legs and arms with a warm napkin at least twice a week. Excellent for dry, flaky skin.

You can improve their texture too -- flaky dry arms can be made silky by using a loofah (a rough, hand glove available in the pharmacy or supermarket.) Wet the glove with soap and water and rub it using a circular motion on both arms and legs. This, besides revving blood circulation, also removes dead, flaky skin; making your skin smooth and supple.

Oil your body after a bath -- spreading baby oil all over your arms and legs, including your feet and toes. Then, towel dry. This keeps your skin sleek and shiny. Hairy arms and legs look untidy and unkempt. If hair on arms isn't noticeable, leave it alone. Legs should be kept hairless as sweat and dust accumulate, making legs look unkempt.

Your first hair removal experience can be traumatic. Every girl goes through it. I remember once seeing a thirteen year old with horribly bruised legs -- she said she used a razor to remove the unwanted hair! She had seen a friend with gorgeous hair-free legs and decided to shave hers off. Never shave arms and legs as you'll need to do this every third day; and the hair will grow back stubbly and coarse. Waxing is your best bet, as the hair takes at least 3 weeks to regrow.

Looking after your hands and legs should be part of your beauty and bath routine. Use a pumice stone daily on your feet and heels; this helps get rid of dead skin. Soap and detergent, in time, dehydrate the skin, so keep your hands, feet and legs soft and protected using the moisturising lotion I've concocted. Soft, silky smooth legs will be ample reward for your effort !

Perfect smoothener

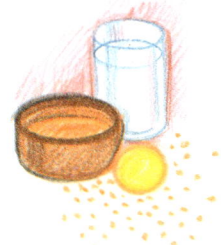

Make a paste of oats, honey, 1/2 tsp. of lemon juice and milk. Apply on arms and legs for 10 minutes before rinsing off.

Wax

NAIL CARE

Nails on hands and feet should be clipped once a fortnight to improve their quality. If you wish to have long nails, make sure they're strong and healthy -- their grooming will be noticed, not their health. After clipping them to a decent length, use an emery board to file them. Never use metal nail files on your fingers; as this can be is hard on them. And never dig into your nails with a nail file. Always use a nail brush to clean your nails.

250 gms. sugar, 1 cup lime juice. Keep this mixture in a heavy pot over a gentle fire and keep stirring till it gets honey brown and sticky. Remove from fire, cool and use when required. Warm it before using by immersing container in a pot of warm water.

Your nails have to grow healthy and strong. A diet comprising a glass of warm milk with one teaspoon of gelatin dissolved is excellent -- drink it till your nails harden and improve.

Nail biting is an irritating habit; besides making the nails look ugly. Lemon juice dabbed on nails will help strengthen them besides being a deterrent, as the nails will be bitter to taste.

You probably love painted nails. But if you apply one polish over the other and leave it for months on end, the school principal, one day, will pull you up; by which time you'll need a blade to remove the build-up of polish. Learn how to apply and remove polish as well as the rudiments of nail care, as, once your nails are damaged, they'll probably never recover.

Say it With Your Eyes

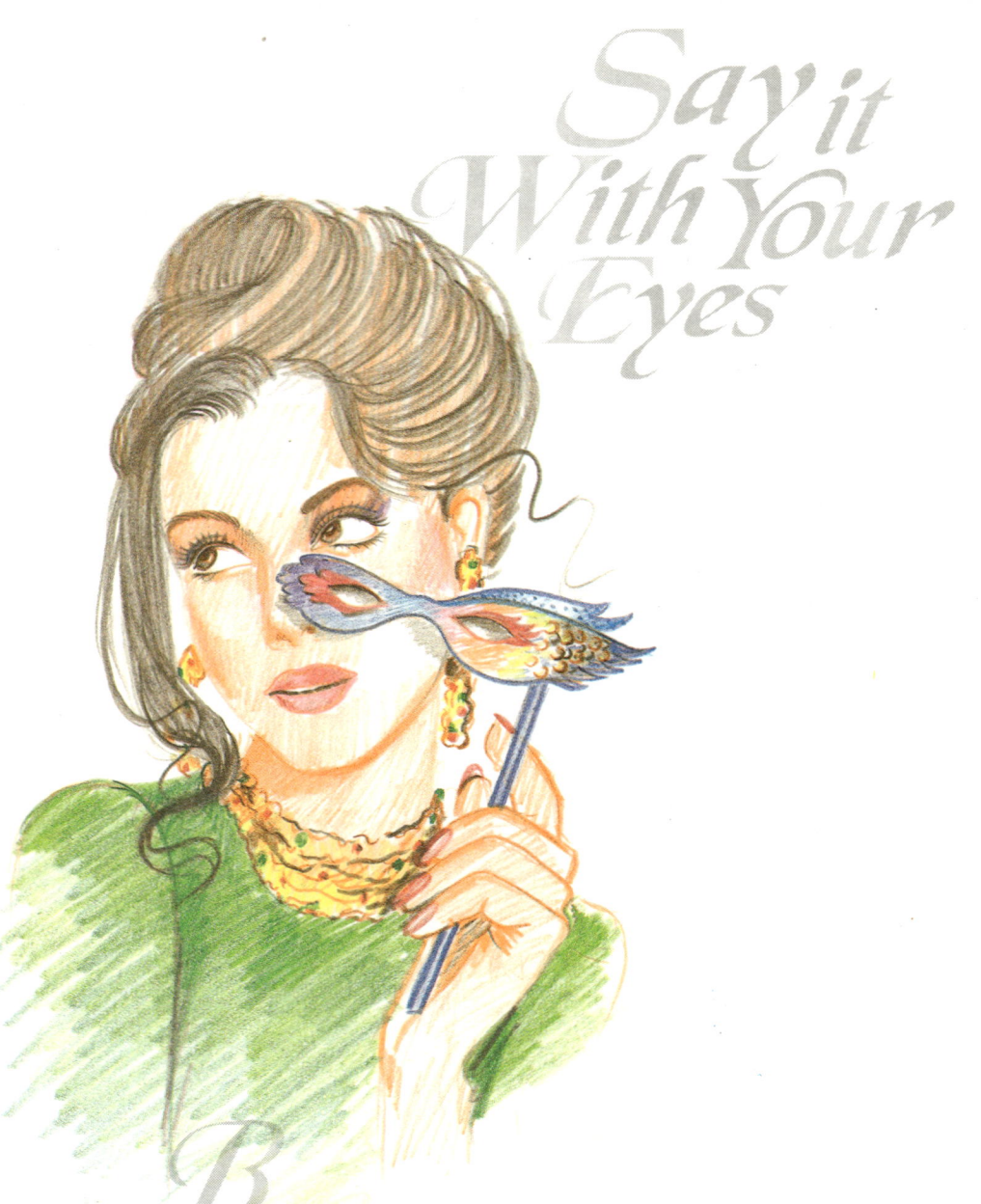

Bright, sparkling eyes are your most shining asset, so look after them! Sleep, fresh air and exercise all help keep your eyes clear and luminous. Spend time in natural light, and when reading and writing, ensure the light is behind or above you; never in front. Study early in the morning rather than late at night; and try to give yourself a break of 15 minutes after every hour of study, using that time to do a few simple eye exercises to soothe them. Blink every few seconds, then cup your eyes in your hands. This will help relax and refresh them.

Your eyebrows frame and define your eyes. This is another area where, without proper guidance, you can err with disastrous results. A cousin, who had eyebrows that met at her nose had razored them off; uncaring about the shape. Imagine the damage she did to her soft features. With the right guidance, she could have saved herself from cosmetic disaster!

Avoid sitting with smokers, especially while studying. Smoking is an irritant ... the nicotine causes the blood vessels in the eyes to constrict, while this coupled with carbon monoxide decreases the blood vessels ability to carry oxygen.

In case you watch television avidly, do so after sunset, in a brightened room. Switch on sidelights which should ideally be placed so that no reflections are caused on the screen. The television, incidentally, should be placed just below eye level. Keep your distance from the television -- 3-4 metres is adequate. And if the movie isn't too riveting, look away occasionally, just for a few seconds.

Cool milk pads relax, cool, and moisturise.

You probably are aware of this... don't read in moving vehicles. Shifting vision can strain the eyes, causing them to weaken and strain.

Crushed mint paste is great for dark circles.

As a child, I used Kajal in my eyes. However late it was, my mother insisted I clean my eyes before sleeping, as she said foreign particles caused weak eyesight. I hated wearing spectacles, so I obeyed her. She dipped cotton wool in rose water and added a little castor oil. This was my eye cleansing lotion and I use it to this day! Castor oil strengthens lashes while rose water cools. Splashing your eyes with tea water also helps. And if you're going through a period of eyestrain, cup your eyes occasionally. It keeps the light away, relieving eye strain. It's important though, to have a diet that is abundantly rich in Vitamins A and C.

Use warm tea bags on your eyes if you wish to take a short break from your books, and chilled tea bags if you want to be up and about again.

So eat plenty of carrots and celery. Nothing, though, rivals carrot juice for your daily dose of Vitamin A!

A small pinch of salt in tap water brightens dull eyes. Bathe them by cupping the palm of your hand.

Sparkling, beautiful eyes are one of the best assets a woman can have. My advice to you: pamper and indulge them unashamedly.

Witch hazel eye pads cool and lighten sore eyes.

EYE EXERCISES

To strengthen vision and keep your eyes looking luminous, exercise them daily.

<> Looking straight at the mirror, make a circular movement with your eyes, first clockwise, then anti-clockwise. Repeat this 8 times.

<> Keeping your head straight and still, look up at the ceiling then down to the floor. Do this rapidly 8 times.

<> Without moving your head, turn your pupil to the extreme right, then to the extreme left. Repeat this 8 times.

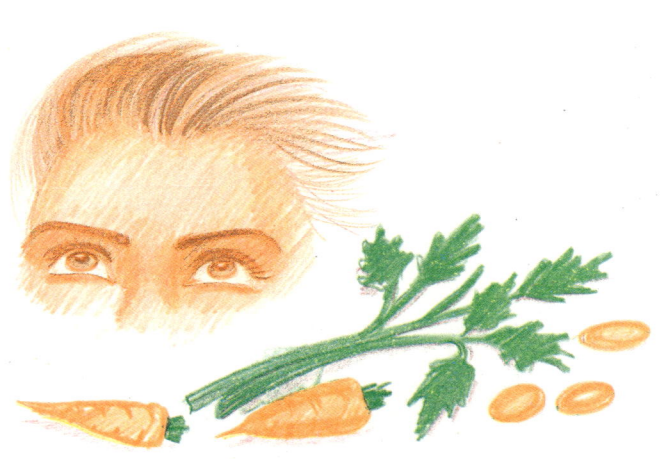

Occasion-al Beauty

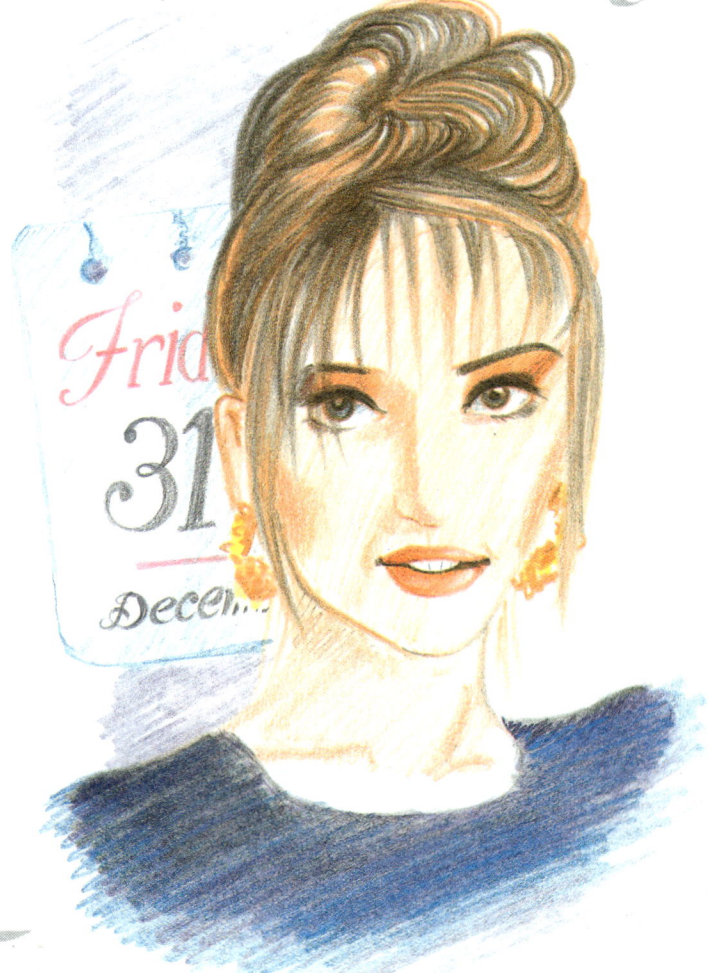

There's always that special occasion - a date, your birthday, your anniversary, a prom or, simply summer holidays when you're winging your way to some place special, for which you'd like to go all out with that little bit of extra effort; and look gorgeous !

SUMMER HOLIDAYS

First, some quick remedies to prepare yourself for that long planned summer break:

Prepare a paste of almond powder and cucumber juice. Add 2 drops of lemon and a pinch of turmeric powder, apply this paste on your face and body to lighten. Oil your hair at least twice a week preceding your departure and use a protein pack like the one I've described.

Besides clipping and filing your nails with an emery board, soften your hands with a daily almond oil massage to strengthen your nails and soften your hands.

To really look and feel sensational, go on a fruit diet for 2 days -- avoid tea, coffee, alcohol and cigarettes. Avoid citrus fruits and avocados. Any other fruit is fine.

Drink light herbal tea, and make it a point to have a minimum of 2 liters of water daily for a few days before leaving. This will help cleanse your body of toxins; as well as give you an incredibly light and buoyant feeling.

You're all set now... all you need to do is pack your bags. Don't forget your beauty box, plastic bottles, a small brush, a mixing bowl and a headband to pull your hair back! And have a great time!

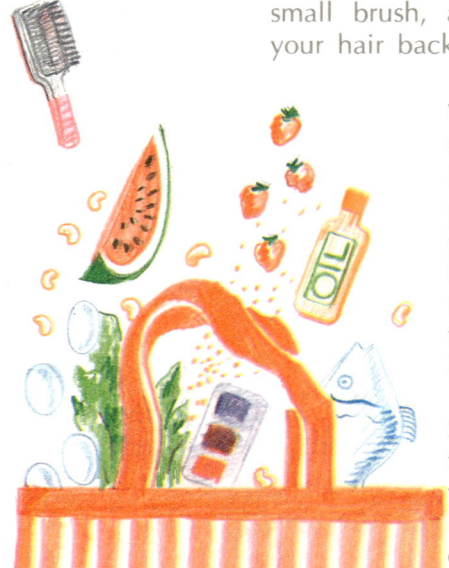

THE NEW YEAR

We've come full circle, and the new year is upon us again. We've had a string of late nights preceding New Years Eve, and we're probably looking worn on this day of hope and resolutions! We've bought a new dress for the occasion; and we'd like to look, in a word ravishing. Take heart... it's possible:

Start gearing yourself for the big day a few days before. First, relax... making sure your clothes and accouterments are clean, ironed and hung for the big day. Next, exfoliate your skin every few days with rice powder, yogurt and honey. If your skin is dry, substitute cream for honey, and almond for rice powder. Exfoliating is a process of scrubbing that rids the body of dead skin and cells. Make sure you scrub the ingredients gently with your fingers into your skin.

Again, every couple of days, before the big day, smoothen your skin to an even tone with chilled honey combined with carrot juice or pulp; this is great as a skin smoothener. Avocado pulp, applied for twenty minutes every alternate day under your eyes will fade dark circles. Apply this for at least a week prior to New Years Eve. Also, make sure you condition your hair to a dramatic gloss with henna and black tea!

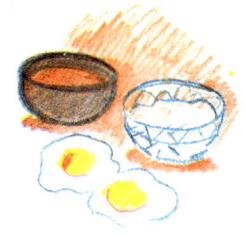

Hair Pack

1 egg, 2 tbsps. yogurt, almond powder, fenugreek powder. Use this hair pack on oiled hair. After shampooing, rinse with vinegar and water.

On New Years Eve itself, start your morning with a cup of "Camomile tea", with just a teaspoon of honey. This, incidentally, is a great nerve calmer!

Exercise for just ten minutes -- nothing gives you quite the kind of 'high' exercise does. Keep it simple -- just five minutes of skipping and five of calisthenics.

You've already kept your eye pack prepared and chilled -- this one made from cucumber and potato juice. Chill it and let it rest on the eyes for at least 10 minutes, making sure you have 2 pillows under your feet and none under your head -- to keep that circulation buzzing. The eye pack should lighten those dark rings.

Use an abundantly rich, special hair pack. Two yolks of egg mixed with one tablespoon of brandy massaged into your scalp and hair for half an hour will give it a never before shine.

Next, treat your face and body to something unabashedly luxurious. Mix together, one tablespoon yogurt, two egg yolks, one tablespoon honey and one tablespoon of almond and oats powder. The mixture should not be too runny. If it is, add more oats. Get into a dry bath tub and rub the mixture on the entire face and body. While the pack dries, you could, perhaps, repeat the eye pack and relax. The body pack is particularly great for nourishing, smoothening, rejuvenating and exfoliating your skin. Once your hair and body pack dry, wash them off with your favorite shampoo and soap. Dry yourself and lather on that lotion!

Now your face: add some rose water to a basin of chilled water and dip your face in the basin, repeating five times. This will freshen and enliven your face. Dab dry and moisturise immediately.

If your hands and feet require a manicure, do this, including the nail polish, in the morning. Choose your make-up carefully; (preferably in the morning, to avoid last minute stress) -- and keep the eyeshadow, blusher, highlighter, mascara, loose powder and perfume ready in a tray. This will ensure that, come evening, you'll feel calm, organised and collected!

If you're not an organised person and you're feeling up to it, I'd go a step further and recommend you have a dress rehearsal the day before, to be really set up and 'together' for the big day.

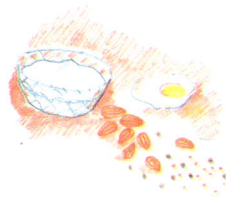

Body pack for Summer and the New Year:

Take two yolks, 1 tbsp. honey and one of yogurt. Mix well before adding a tablespoon of almond and a tablespoon of oats powder. If the mixture is too runny; add more oats. Get into a dry bath tub and rub the mixture on your entire face and body. Leave this to dry for at least 20 minutes. Rinse off.

Now, (and we're still in the morning), dry your hair and set it in your favorite style. Don't leave the shampooing till the evening, as freshly shampooed hair never sets well. Set your hair morning or evening.

Your evening rests on the mood you've been in the whole day, so today, concentrate on yourself -- listening to music that enlivens you, meeting the people who give you a high, and eating fruits and salads in abundance. Flake out in the afternoon - a short nap will keep you going for hours at night. Believe me; you feel good, you'll look good.

Above all, think positive: making a whole lot of impossible-to-meet New Year resolutions will aid that positive 'mindset'. Start the year off right, and you'll probably meet your resolutions at least halfway!

Do Your Hands and Legs Need a Hand?

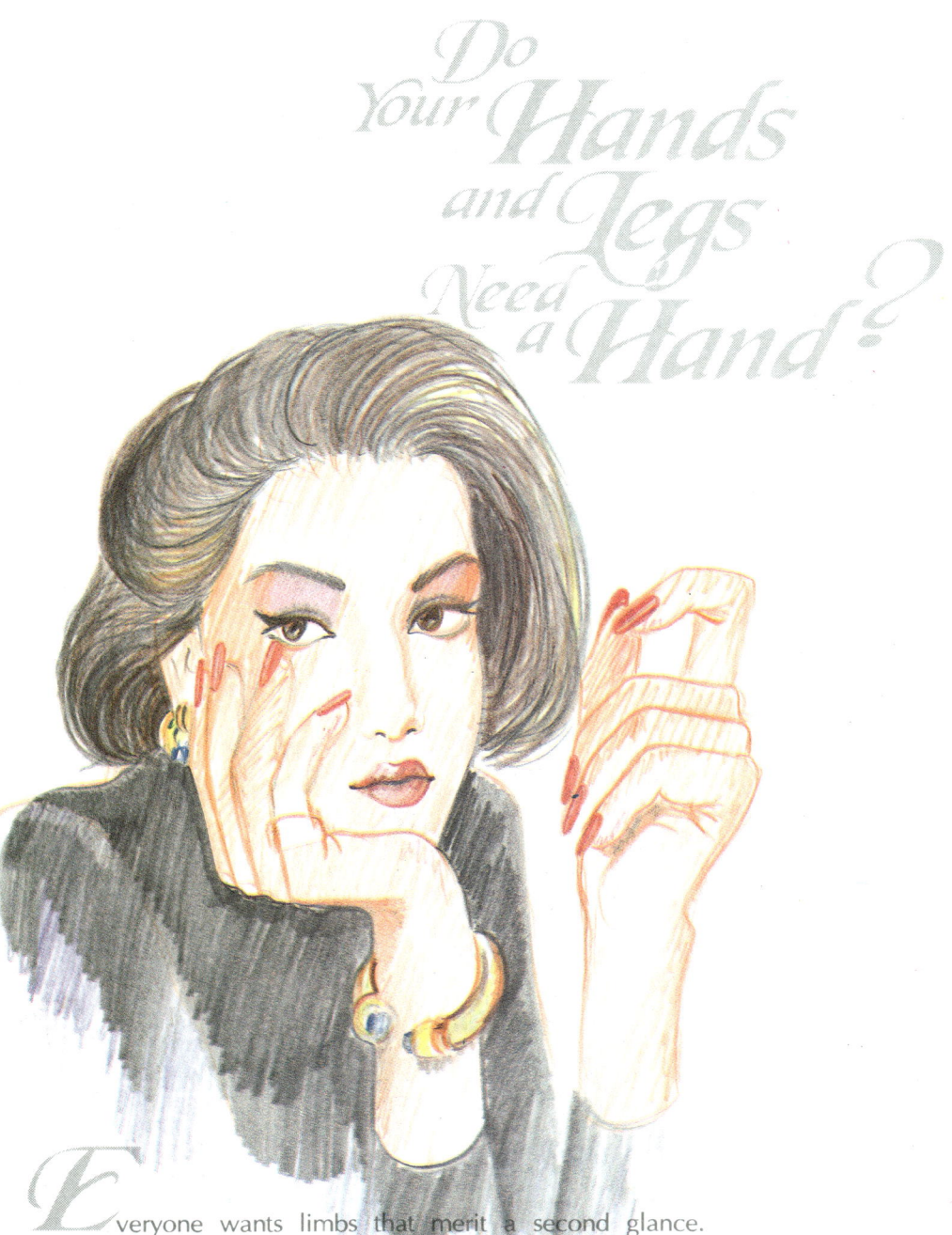

Everyone wants limbs that merit a second glance. Without exercise and a regular toning routine, your arms and legs become soft and flabby. This is easily overcome by simple exercise routines like rotating the arms clockwise and anti-clockwise at least ten times for each arm.

Another simple exercise: Hold a heavy book in each palm and spread arms sideways at shoulder level. Bend elbow bringing book to shoulder and return to starting position. Do this ten times. Both these exercises will help tone and shape your arms.

Unimaginably long, sleek legs are not so easy to come by, but you can work at it: Stand straight, resting your hands on a chair back. Swing the right leg as high as possible and bring back to position without touching the ground. Do this continuously 10 times. Now work on the other leg. This reduces thigh flab besides giving you a long-legged look. For strong, well shaped legs, walk on your toes for one minute and then rest on your ankles. Repeat this ten times.

It isn't enough to have shapely arms and legs. You need to improve their texture: flaky, dry legs and arms need to be stimulated every day. Use a loofah. Wet and rub soap on it and, with a circular motion, use it both on arms and legs for 1 minute on each limb. This improves blood circulation and removes flaky dead skin, making it smooth, shiny and supple.

Every four days make a paste of oats, adding one teaspoon of lemon juice and milk. Mix into a paste and apply it over arms and legs. Rinse off after five minutes. Always oil your body after your bath. When your body is wet, spread baby oil all over arms and legs -- including feet and toes. Then towel dry. This keeps the skin shiny and smooth.

Hair on legs and arms looks untidy and ungroomed. If the hair on your arms is not too noticeable, leave it. Legs though, should be kept hairless, as sweat and dust accumulate, making them look unkempt. Waxing is your best bet. You won't need to bother about removing your hair again for another three weeks. Never shave arms and legs, as you will be doing this every 3rd day. Besides, the hair will grow back stubbly and coarse.

Caring for your arms and legs should be part of your regular beauty care regimen. Soaps and detergents are drying, so always keep your feet and hands protected by

Home-made Moisturiser

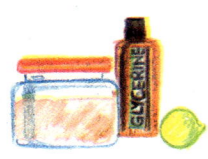

Mix well 6 tsps. of petroleum jelly, 2 tsp. of glycerine and 1/2 a tsp. of lemon juice. Apply all over arms and legs. Remember to include your feet. Then take a warm napkin and gently dab the skin. This is an excellent cream for dry skin.

Wrinkled Knees

Rub cleansing cream or fresh cream on knees with a few drops of lemon juice. Leave on for 10 minutes; then rinse off with ground or crushed lemon peel.

a home-made moisturiser based on petroleum jelly and glycerine. Do this before going to bed. Also, scrub your feet every day with a pumice stone. This helps scour dead skin from your heels and feet, ensuring the skin remain soft and supple.

Make sure your knees aren't dark and wrinkled even if you were punished and made to kneel when you were a child! If you were, make amends now by preparing my rather complicated but effective paste for dark, wrinkled, knees! The orange peel lightens and smoothens, Vitamin E or almond oil helps iron out crinkles, cream too, bleaches and softens while honey works as a softener and cleanser. If you can't make the paste, make sure you keep using oil after your bath or before retiring at night. The paste though, is a great knee smoothener.

CARING FOR NAILS

Like your hair, your nails reflect the way you feel, highlighting poor nutrition, an unhealthy lifestyle, health problems, nervousness and shoddy nail care.

Interestingly, in summer, your nails grow faster than in winter. Vital to good looking, growing nails, though, is protein. Brewers Yeast, almonds, eggs, apricots and liver are supposed to be good nail food.

To spur growth, massage your nails with warm almond oil and push the cuticles back daily. At night, before retiring, dip your nails in lemon juice or vinegar. These are nail strengtheners, helping your nails grow faster.

To keep nails from breaking and splitting avoid using detergents and household chemicals. Wear gloves when rinsing clothes as water and chemicals weaken the nails.

Dial the phone with a pencil instead of your fingers and pick things up with your fingers, not nails.

Keep your nails smoothly filed so they don't get jagged edges that get caught in clothes. Do not remove polish every day as acetone dries and weakens nails. You

Knees (contd...)

Take orange peel and dry it in the sun or oven. Grind it into a fine powder. Mix 1 tsp. of this with 1 tsp. almond powder, 1 tsp. cream and 1 tsp. honey to make a smooth paste.

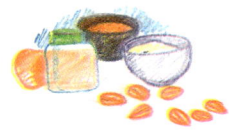

Apply this beauty paste to your knees and leave it on for 30 minutes. Now, for 5 minutes, keep massaging the knee with the paste. Rinse with cool water. Make sure you dry it thoroughly and apply vitamin E or almond oil on the knees regularly as this helps smoothen the skin.

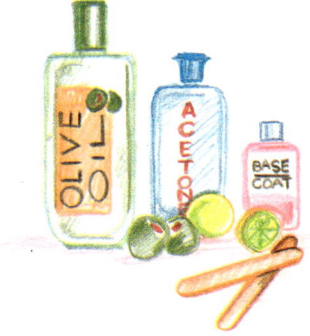

could add a drop of lemon juice and olive oil to the acetone to prevent your nails from drying out.

The base coat is an essential before applying polish, as besides holding the colored polish, it also protects the nail plate from absorbing colour.

In-growing toe nails are extremely painful, as anyone who has suffered will tell you. They develop due to shoes that are too narrow or tight, clumsy cutting or injury. In rare cases, it can become a perpetual problem.

Cutting the corners of the nails back into the nail grooves often leads to ingrowing toe nails. These are mainly caused because the nail edge grows into the skin, which then folds back over it.

Cutting your nails straight across helps. Do not dig into the corner as you may inflame the skin. Insert an orange stick (available at the pharmacy) in at the corner of the nail and gently fill the corner. Don't dig deep. This treatment gently lifts the nail from under the skin improving it's condition. If you find the problem untractable, visit a doctor as he will have a solution.

Do not cut your nails in a hurry; cut them immediately after a bath as, once softened, you don't need to apply force. Toe nails are tough nuts to crack and if you find, even after a bath, that they haven't softened, dip your feet in warm water for 10 minutes.

Never shape nails while cutting with a nail cutter; clip them straight across and round them off with an emery (and not a metal) file.

Good looking nails don't happen overnight. They require attention and care. The effort is well worth it. For, if your nails are ungroomed, it has a telling effect on all of you. I like to think that well groomed nails gives you the finishing touch; that final gloss. So do take the trouble to polish up those tips!

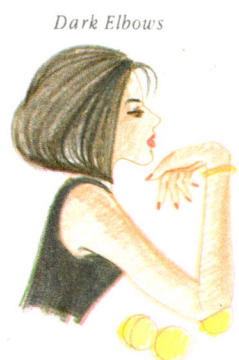

Dark Elbows

Lighten your elbows by leaning them on fresh lemon halves.

Tone that Body

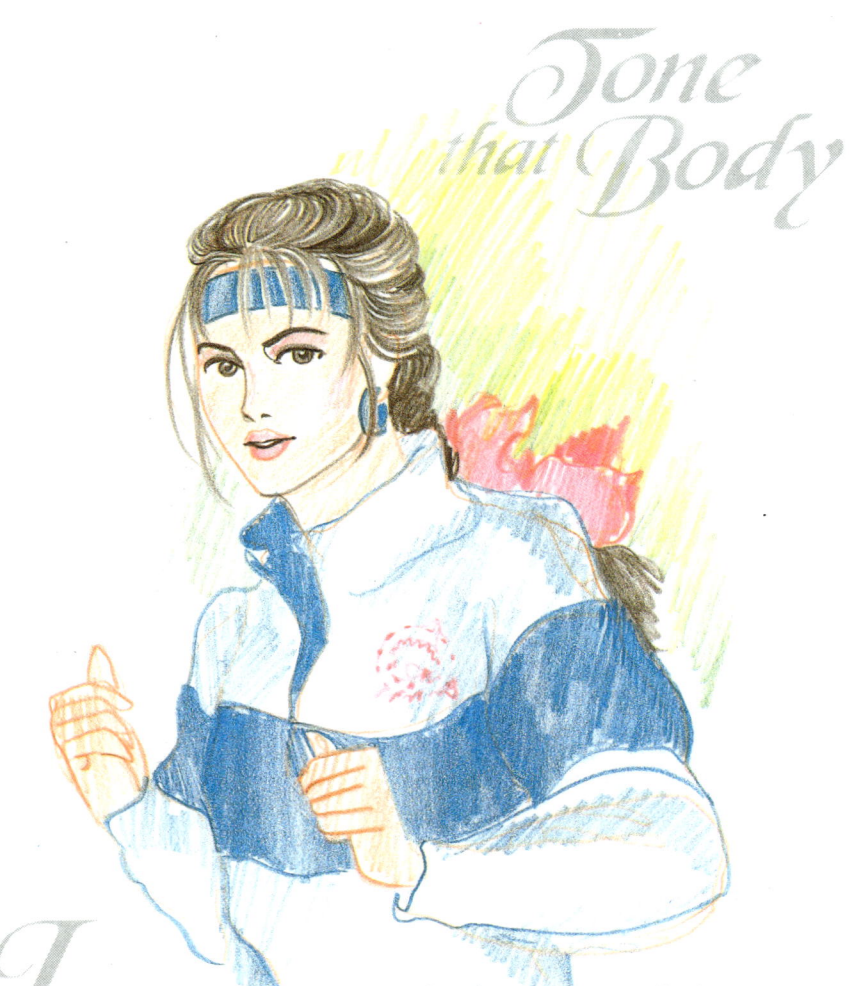

Let me stress the importance of exercise above all else. It firms muscles, moves joints, and makes you supple. It improves circulation by increasing the intake of oxygen. And, most importantly, it relaxes the mind, delaying the aging process.

Exercise is not boring. Quite the contrary, it's your attitude that makes it so. It's important to find an exercise that blends with your lifestyle, your system and your needs. Calisthenics was the rage, and now it's aerobics. There'll always, of course, be changing fads, but I advise you to steer clear of what is 'vogue-ish' and select something that suits your temperament.

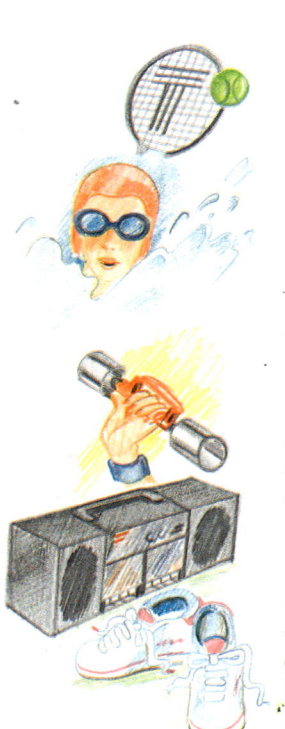

Exercise does not merely alter your weight; it helps to tone and tighten the body and restore firmness. You'll notice the inches falling off and your weight whittling -- this, of course, is the toning process.

It's important, at the outset, to mentally prepare yourself to enjoy the exercise. Select a spot you like, perhaps by a window or near a favorite plant, and fix a particularly unrushed time of day, or you'll never do justice to the exercise. That takes care of your mood and time. Now lift your mood further by investing in a beautiful leotard or track suit, an exercise mat (it isn't advisable to work out on carpets as carpet threads can cause nose and throat irritations). Then, switch on your favorite music, so that you exercise at a pace and beat you enjoy -- and you're all set!

Exercise, if well done, raises and maintains your pulse rate above normal while a fresh supply of oxygen courses through your system. Observe a basic rule - exhale while the body is bent and compressed and inhale as you stretch or straighten. In case you're over 35, get yourself medically examined before you rush into an exercise program. And always stop when you feel fatigued or breathless. With time, this will happen with decreasing frequency.

Now let's get down to the different types of exercise and how they help us. There's something out there for everybody: you can walk, jog, run, cycle, skip, and skate. You can play tennis, badminton or squash. You can swim, skate, or ride; You can do yoga, gymnastics or weight training.

Walking is a great body toner, especially for the foot and calf muscles. Always walk energetically as lethargic walking, or, dragging your feet is ineffective.

Jogging strengthens the calves and exercises the heart and lungs. It especially exercises the hips, knee and ankle joints. Never start jogging without a few warm - up exercises. And make sure your jogging shoes are well padded and comfortable.

An advise. It is important to know your potential. Don't rush to doing vigorous jogging. Start with brisk walks and then graduate to jogging. When you finish your jog and have sweated do not forget to towel off your sweat.

Cycling is a good, vigorous exercise that tones the buttocks, and the thigh and calf muscles. It increases the flexibility of your knees and ankles.

Skipping is excellent for the entire body. Rest in between, if you need to, for at least a minute, and once again, warm up first!

Swimming, too, exercises all your muscles. Water is the perfect exercise medium as it supports your weight without any risk of strain. The various strokes use different muscles, so it's good to alternate them for best effect. The crawl tightens abdominal muscles, slims inner thighs and upper arms. The side stroke tones waist, legs and arms, while the butterfly exercises the chest, thigh, arm and shoulder muscles.

Yoga is best for suppleness and as a relaxant. It alleviates tension like nothing else does. Yogasanas, or yogic exercises should be done under instruction, as forcing certain postures exerts an unreasonable strain on your muscles.

Weight training is a good way to firm and tone areas that other exercises neglect to stress i.e. your upper arms and inner thighs.

Relaxation is the best tonic for your body. Never confuse sleeping with relaxation. Relaxation is a state of mind when your eyes are open and your mind is free and uncluttered from thoughts. Just once a day, get away from the family, television, books and music and just lie in the garden or by the window thinking, literally, nothing. I find it revitalizes me more than 7 hours of the deepest sleep.

Relaxation is also energizing. And energy generates more energy. The more you exercise, and the more completely you relax, the better you will feel.

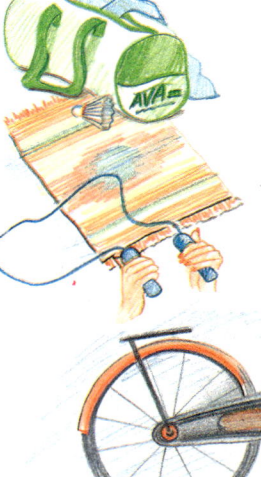

Once you have started on your exercise programme you will notice a radiance on your face and a spring in your walk. And you'll probably be an exercise addict for life!

YOGA: FOR BODY AND SOUL

YOGA, an Indian import, is fast becoming popular due to its calming, energizing effect on both body and mind. You can practice yoga at any age, it's never too late to adopt this discipline. Increasingly, as the pace of life quickens, people around the globe are finding solace in yoga.

A remarkable feature of yoga is that, unlike other vigorous exercises, yoga is slow and disciplined. The body is never forced into a position, but is phased into it gradually, as it develops agility and control.

Yoga can correct recurring health disorders such as indigestion, menstrual problems and colds. Slow, serene and pleasant, yogasanas enhance your face, transforming, incredibly, the way you look. The deep breathing asanas in yoga relax while creating self-awareness and the muscle flexing required in other asanas are scientifically designed to tone, invigorate and heal.

Yoga corrects your breathing technique. Its controlled, deep breathing helps remove waste from the lungs clearing your body of impurities and brings a healthy glow to the skin. Yet another breathing technique called 'alternate breathing', that is, breathing through one nostril and then the other, is said to compose the mind and clear stuffed nasal passages.

Yoga cures insomnia too, as the stretched positions, held for a while, allow sleep to come more easily. It also helps cure smoking. Die - hard smokers, I've heard, have reformed with deep breathing asanas. Expecting mothers practice Yoga to ease labour and you can delay lines and sagging skin through the "Lion Roar", a toning exercise derived from Yoga: Cleanse the face thoroughly, spread a smooth film of vitamin E oil in an upward direction over the neck and face, including eyes. Open your mouth wide and keep the tongue stretched out, hanging downwards. Keep this position as long as you can; then relax. Repeat five times daily.

Yoga also incorporates meditation techniques that help the body relax and feel as if it is floating on air. This is a contented state of being, which, I assure you, even sleep cannot achieve. Yoga, always practiced on an empty stomach, requires a well ventilated room. Ideally, wear clothes like loose cotton trousers or shorts and loose T shirts.

However, it is absolutely essential that yoga be professionally taught and not practiced by reading a manual or looking at pictures.

Once you've discovered an exercise regimen that suits you, half your battles won. Go for it, for no matter what else you do, if you're flabby and your body's untoned; you'll never reach your great looking potential!

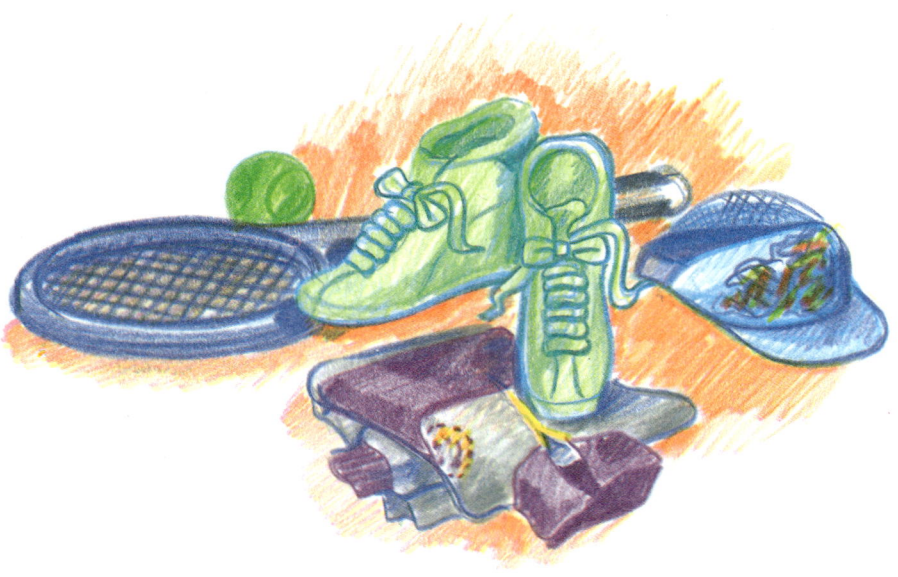

Facing Wrinkles

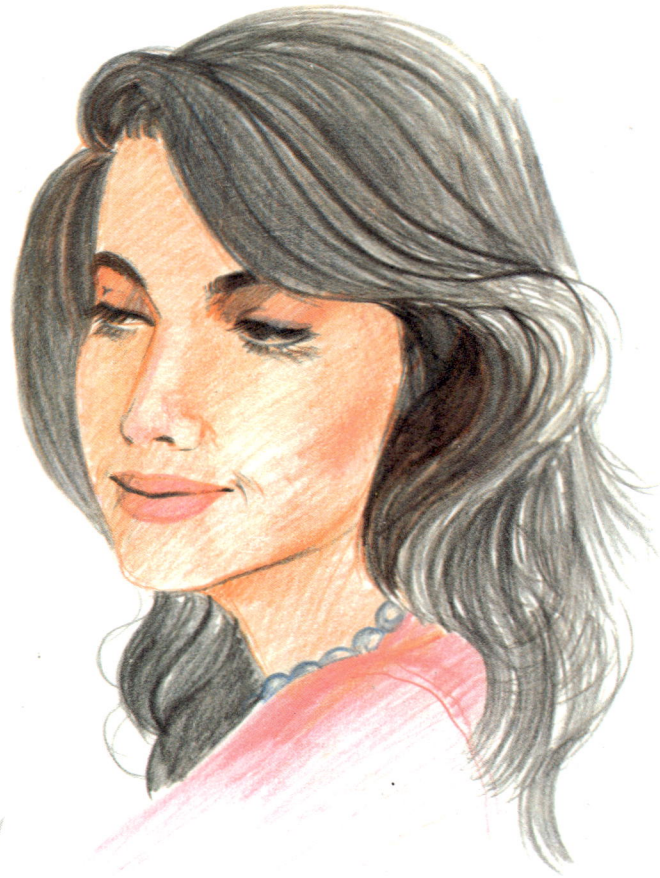

A ge gracefully. Even though your skin has its own chronological age which may or may not coincide with yours. There are many environmental and genetic factors that accelerate and retard the aging process. Line-erasing and face-lifting techniques which promise to subtract years from the face and restore it to it's former bloom don't always work. Your age tends to creep up on you slowly, indelibly, revealing itself through your face.

Sophia Loren, the beautiful and mature actress, once said: "Coming to terms with age" is one of the best achievements of your life. There's a lovely charm in aging gracefully, so don't fight it. Certainly, there's nothing as ungracious and ungainly as a middle-aged woman who tries to pass herself off as a teenager.

I, in fact, would advise you to follow the maxim, 'Look your age'. You need to mentally and physically come to terms with age. The eye shadow or lipstick that looked good on you at 20 may not suit you after 20 years. Nor the hairstyle; and certainly not your clothes. This is because your skin tone and texture, hair colour and features all change gradually with the passage of time. If at any stage you've become 'fixed in time', that is, your make-up and the way you look is stale and hackneyed; then it's time you consulted a professional makeup expert for fresh ideas and inspiration.

Age can be broken up into three brackets:

The teens: A time for experimentation. Skin care routines learned now will stand you in good stead for the rest of your life. Teenagers, typically, spend hours in front of the mirror scrutinising their features, and teenage girls tend to change their hair styles to transform their image very often.

The 20s: A time of confidence. You have the experience to know which make-up and hair style are right for you. Skin care towards the end of this decade is particularly important, as about this time, the first few lines begin to appear.

The 30s and above: A time for boldness. A complete switch of hair colour and make-up can rejuvenate you. Your body is probably in as good a shape as it was in the 20s, and if it is not, diet and exercise can help. Entertaining at home and going out give you opportunities to wear good clothes and great make-up to complement them.

Beauty lies in making the most of your natural looks. It requires an understanding of your physical drawbacks

Stress combatant

Prepare a paste of mint leaves and almonds. Mix well in warm water and apply over the entire body. Make a henna paste mixed in warm tea leaves: apply this to the scalp. Leave till body and scalp dry. Rinse them off with warm water. These body and hair packs are refreshing and soothing to the nerves.

Use eye gel regularly

and doing what you can to overcome them. This is in fact one of the most fascinating aspects of beauty care - seeing yourself clearly and enjoying what you see. For only you can help yourself realise your beauty potential.

Exaggerated facial expressions, anxiety and age are the main cause of wrinkles and worry lines. The following facial exercises will help ease lines and facial features:

The most important muscles, from the beauty viewpoint are the zygonatius muscles which extend across the cheeks from the temples to the mouth corners. They keep the contours of the face firm and go a long way in determining facial features and expressions. Chewing strengthens these muscles. Laughing and smiling also help as they pull the corners of the mouth in an upward direction, preventing the face from sagging.

If you decide to start exercising your facial muscles, maintain a certain momentum, as if you stop, the muscles will slacken again. Face exercises should be done in private, so, if possible, close your door and take a comfortable position in front of your dressing table mirror. Cleanse your skin before beginning; applying a tonic and a thin film of vitamin E oil to your face and neck. This is important in keeping your skin supple as skin should never be stretched when dry. Tie your hair back, so your face is free and unencumbered.

Forehead: Lift the forehead, forcing it upwards. Keep in position for a second then release. Do this ten times.

Crows feet: Open eyes wide for a second then relax. Repeat this ten times.
Under-the-eye wrinkles: Open the eye wide and look upwards then downwards. Repeat this ten times.

Eyes: The entire eye requires a clockwise and anti-clockwise eyeball movement. It is both relaxing and toning.

Nose: Twist the mouth to its maximum -- to the right side first and then to the left. Keep in the twisted position for a second.

The mouth, cheek and jaw: Open your mouth to it's maximum and stick your tongue out till you feel it hurts. This exercise tones the entire jaw and mouth area.

Neck: Throw your neck back to the maximum and, with the help of the lower teeth, blow out air. Repeat this exercise ten times.

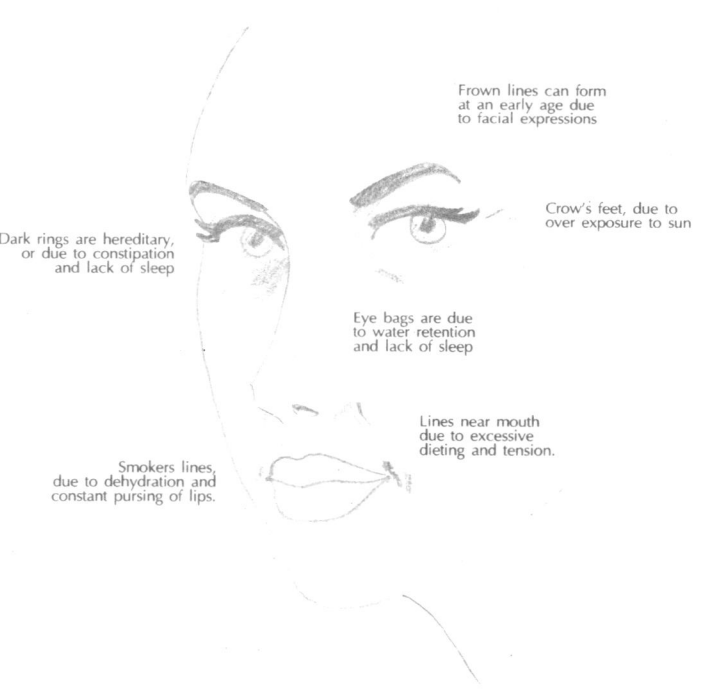

In between each exercise, inhale and exhale. Besides toning your skin this also adds colour to your complexion.

Wrinkles around the eyes are to a great extent due to age. They may also be due to excessive skin dryness or exposure to sun without proper sunglasses. The lack of sebaceous glands in this area are also one of the major reasons for the skin losing it's smoothness. Frequent lubrication is very important.

Facial Oils

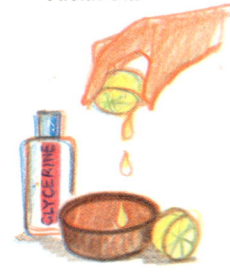

2 tsp. Vit E oil or 1/2 tsp. glycerine with a drop of lime juice or 2 capsules Vitamin E oil combined with 2 drops glycerine

Apply an eye oil or gel with the ring finger. Pat the oil gently without actually massaging the eye areas as this does more harm than good by stretching delicate skin. Removing eye makeup is essential. Make-up left overnight will dry up the delicate skin around the eyes. Simply dab eye make-up remover on damp cotton pads against the eye then wipe gently outwards. Reverse the pad. Hold against the same eye. This cleanses and moisturizes your skin.

The throat and neck are the first places to show lines and wrinkles partly because of the scarcity of sebaceous glands in this area and poor posture. Skin should always be lubricated around the neck as throat lines start to form very early (as young as the mid-twenties unless the skin is kept well lubricated)! Massage a rich, lubricating cream in with the knuckles from the base of the throat to the chin.

You can't beat age, but by following an unfaltering beauty regimen, you can certainly meet it head-on !

PREPARE FOR MENOPAUSE

Menopause is the great leveler. All women, from every walk of life face it between their 50s and 60s. This is around the period when your menstrual cycle comes to a halt and pregnancy is no longer possible.

Speaking to several women on their experiences, one gathers that a major problem that needs overcoming is the lack of support demonstrated by family members. This causes even greater depression than that caused by the hormonal cycle.

Though menopause has many symptoms, the major ones are insomnia, hot flushes, vaginal dryness, allergies or itchiness, depression, lethargy and irritability. Occasionally, menopause may be marked by constipation, gas and pigmentation.

Some women, the chosen few, sail through menopause effortlessly, enjoying life as much as they did in their 30s, while some get sensitive and wary socially, going into their shells. Then of course there are those women who become insecure about their appearance. Menopause isn't an easy time. The skin texture thickens, and stray hair might begin to appear on the cheeks, chin and upper lip. A full, lush head of hair might begin to lose its buoyancy and lustre.

Take yourself in hand. This is the time to strike back, not buckle under and cry. All you need is a regular beauty routine that you can adhere to at home. And occasionally, do indulge yourself by visiting a beauty parlor.

Meditation and yoga should be incorporated as part of your beauty routine...to improve the quality of your life. I have been practising meditation for 15 years, and I know, first hand that it eases and clarifys the mind, making life calmer, more meaningful and yes, more efficient. Yoga, besides being a great body and muscle toner; peps circulation.

Then, of course there's Hormone Replacement Therapy. When, during menopause, a womans ovaries stop making oestrogen, it causes the skin to thicken and excessive facial hair. Hormone replacement tablets should be taken strictly under a doctors supervision ...women I know who've done this have had a tremendous zest for life and buoyancy through menopause. There are of course, women, who would shy away from such aids and let nature take it's course.

I recommend the following beauty tips that will go a long way towards you looking and feeling great: Massage your face well with rich oils as the skin tends to dry out at this stage. Use any of the oils I've described liberally, using the back of your hand to massage your face and neck. After a good 5 minutes of massaging, take a warm steam towel and steam the face several times so that the treatment penetrates into your skin. You can repeat the oil treatment weekly.

You can also apply the oil generously on the whole body, 15 minutes before a warm shower. Or, the oils could be applied to your hands and feet as it keeps them soft, supple and smooth; eliminating all traces of dryness.

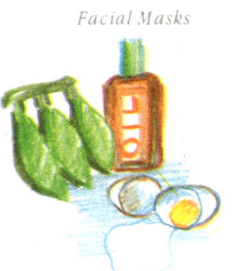

Facial Masks

1/2 tsp. banana,
1 capsule Vitamin E
or 1/2 tsp. Almond Oil,
1 tsp. well beaten egg white.
Leave till firm;
rinse off with cold water.
or
1 Cup almond or oats
powder,
2 tbsp. almond or olive oil
. 2 tbsp. honey,
2 tbsp. milk.
or
1/4 tsp. onion juice,
1/2 tsp. cream
and 1/2 tsp. honey.

Hair Oil for Scalp

*2 tbsp. almond oil
and
1 tbsp. castor oil*

Hair Pack

*2 tbsp. yogurt,
1 tbsp. honey,
and 2 eggs*

Follow the oil treatment with a facial mask and a facial and body scrub at least once a week. Relax with some soothing eye-pads while the mask is on.

Now tackle your hair. It may be dyed, colored or natural; all it needs is a good, warm oil massage twice a week to make it lustrous and bouncy. Hair packs and the bone marrow treatment I've described in the chapter on hair also help.

Drink loads of camomile tea to keep your nerves calm and prevent water retention (another problem faced during menopause).

But above all, live life to the fullest and keep smiling!

Eye Sootheners

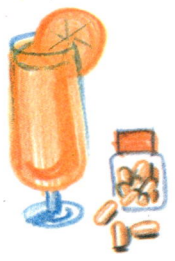

*Use cotton pads dipped
in Orange Juice and
1 capsule Vitamin E oil
or
pulped raw potato
mixed with
1 tsp. Vitamin E oil,
especially good
for crowfeet.*

Highlight on: Hair

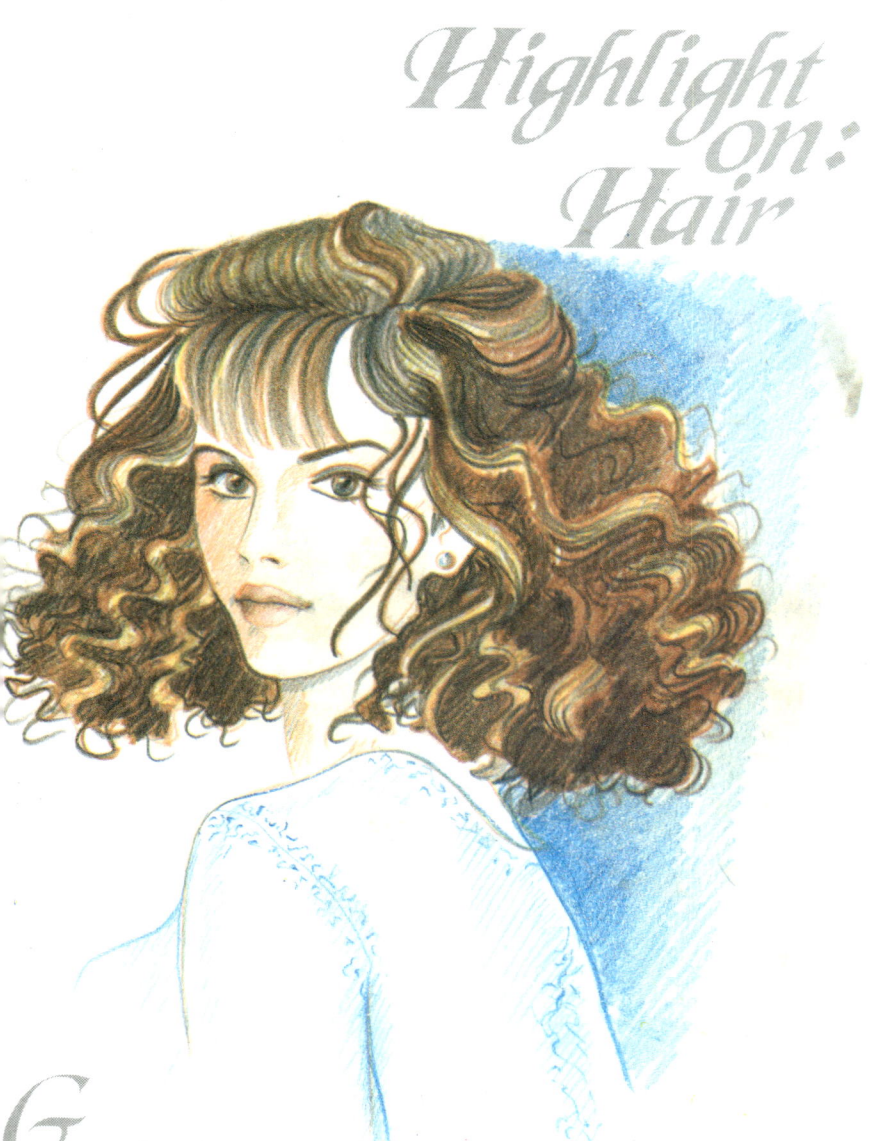

Glossy, luxurious, rapunzel hair can be yours for the asking. Your hair today is under constant onslaught: bleaches, hair dyes, heated rollers, wind, cold, sun, air conditioning, and chlorine in pools all effect the condition of your hair and scalp. Sunlight is particularly harmful as it causes split ends, besides making oily hair oilier and dry hair drier. I'd recommend a weekly treatment or warm oil massage for everybody - regardless of hair type or style. You need

Dull, Lifeless Hair

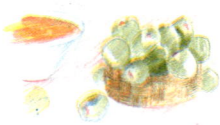

Mix 1/4 cup of green olive oil and 1 cup of honey. Shake vigorously. Allow the mixture to steep for a day or two. Massage into scalp and comb through carefully. Cover your head with a plastic bag, making it air tight so that body heat accelerates penetration. Leave for 30 minutes. Shampoo and rinse.

Beat two eggs, whilst adding 1 tbsp. olive oil, 1 tbsp glycerine and 1 teaspoon cider vinegar. Apply after first shampoo and leave on for 15-30 minutes. Rinse well. If you must, shampoo again. A protein restorer for all types of hair.

Dry Hair

Beat 1 egg, 1 tbsp. vinegar, and 2 tbsp. vegetable oil just before using. Massage into scalp, combing evenly through hair. After 15 minutes, shampoo and rinse. This helps moisturise and lubricate dry scalp and hair. This is not unlike mayonnaise, which is great, in itself, for dry hair.

to massage you hair with your fingertips, rubbing the ingredients gently into the hair partings. This movement draws oxygenated blood to your hair roots, increasing their nourishment. and giving your hair added gloss and life. If your hair cuticle is damaged, a steam towel wrap helps the pores open to absorb oil. For problem hair, use a massage or treatment that addresses your particular problem, every two days.

Not unlike plants, hair roots require nourishment and good circulation; achieved easily via a diet rich in iodine, iron and Vitamin B complex. Foods rich in iron are liver, meat, green vegetables and egg yolk. Remember, hair is made from a form of protein, so a protein-rich diet can work wonders. Make a conscious effort to eat, apart from salads -- eggs, fish, nuts, fresh fruits, cottage cheese and a minimum of eight glasses of water a day. Good supplements are Brewers Yeast powder in juice, soup or water (at least 1 tbsp of yeast powder) or, 2 tablets taken before meals. You could even add 'vegemite' a tasty yeast extract to juices and soups. Wheatgerm and liver tablets too, are effective. As is the B complex group, in the form of Brewers Yeast, wheatgerm, or liver tablets.

Besides this, your diet needs to be finetuned to your hair type. If your hair is greasy, cut down on fried food and fat. If dry, add two tablespoons of salad oil to your regular meals. This, combined with plenty of fresh air, sleep, exercise and a regular hair care regimen will do the trick!

Shampoo is derived from the word, Champua, which means, to rub. Shampoo your hair only with a mild shampoo, as this allows you more than two shampoos a week. Strong shampoos reduce the natural oils in the scalp causing it to feel flaky and dry, so if you're using one, I suggest you dilute it with water. Use luke warm or cold water, finally rinsing with vinegar or lemon juice as this, besides adding a sparkle, helps counter oiliness. If your hair is oily, keep away from sugar and chocolates. Do not use a hair dryer, instead use an electric fan; as hair dryers result in open pores and greasy scalps. Also, steer clear of bath soap on your hair. Bath soap, being alkaline, removes the natural acid mantle of the scalp. Create your own natural conditioning shampoo by adding an egg and 1 tablespoon gelatin, both proteins, to your regular shampoo. If you need a quick conditioner, add yogurt to dry hair, leave it for 15 - 20 minutes and wash it off with an egg shampoo. Remember, conditioners are applied to the hair after rinsing the shampoo off thoroughly. Keep the conditioner on for 5-7 minutes.

One of my favorite shampoos and conditioners is one I've formulated wholly from egg. The yolk is the shampoo; rub it on your hair till it foams. You'll require the yolk of three eggs for shoulder length hair. Rinse this off. For the conditioner, froth the white till it's stiff and forms peaks. Apply, and comb through hair. Rinse it off after ten minutes.

Do you exercise regularly? Just 10 minutes a day touching your toes or skipping helps the body function well and peps blood circulation. It's important, too, to sleep for a continuous 7-8 hours every night. Afternoon naps don't count, they'd never compensate for a night of uninterrupted sleep!

Dry Hair (contd...)

Massage hot oil into scalp and keep on overnight. The next morning, rub lemon and vinegar into scalp. Wash hair with 2 tbsps. shampoo that's been whisked with 1 egg and one cup of water. The last rinse-the juice of a lemon in a cup of hot water. Continue this treatment once a week for three months, then fortnightly for the next two months.

Brush your hair daily as brushing brings the oil coating to the surface of the scalp. Always brush hair in even movements from scalp to hair tips. Daily brushing clears clogged pores, relaxes the head and relieves tension. For added bounce and gloss, throw your hair forward and brush it, again, from your scalp to the hair ends. If your hair is fragile, gently massage 1/2 cup of castor oil into your scalp. Comb through. You could wrap a steaming hot towel around your head for 30 minutes before shampooing, to enable the oil to seep. Hair grows faster at night,

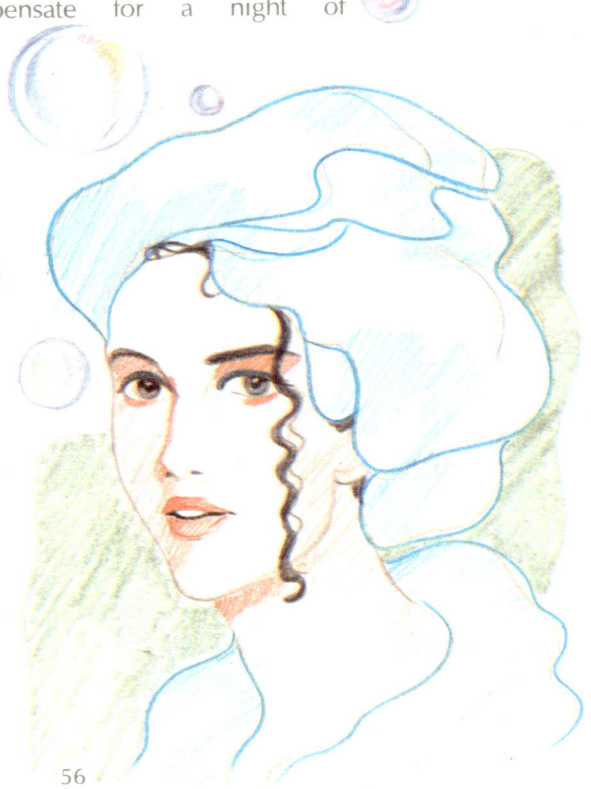

Oily Hair

Gently clean your scalp with a cotton handkerchief wrapped around oats. Or, spread the oats in your scalp, gently massage and then take a dry napkin to clear your hair of oats.

Dandruff

Mix 2 tbsps. cider vinegar with 6 tbsps. of hot water. Part and dab on scalp. Tie a scarf over head and sleep. Next morning, shampoo. The last rinse should consist of 3 tbsps vinegar to one cup hot water. Dry thoroughly and repeat twice weekly for 3 months.

A sugar and lemon scrub on the hair helps. If this doesn't work leave on 4 tsp of warmed olive oil mixed with 1 1/2 tsp. of lemon juice overnight. Shampoo, finally rinsing with vinegar diluted in warm water followed by a cool shower.

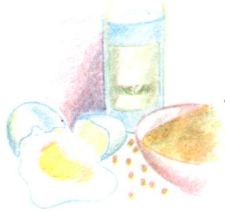

Apply 1 tsp. of fenugreek powder with one egg on scalp. Leave for 20 minutes and wash off with shampoo, followed by a vinegar rinse.

so, castor, olive or almond oil applied at night is more effective. For 'greater glory', you could, the next morning, wrap your hair in hot towels to steam and open your pores. This will enable the oil to seep further.

If you panic every time you see a few hairs on your comb or brush, have a cup of herbal tea (camomile is great) and relax. The average life of a hair is about 5 years, and normal hair loss is at least 60 per day, so, you're bound to see some fallen hair. More than this, though, is abnormal, and usually due to influenza, anxiety, dandruff, childbirth, hormonal changes, sudden shock or antibiotics. Use my specially formulated hair oil, or bone marrow treatment; the recipes of both have been included. I've applied these treatments successfully on my family and friends. Both recipes were developed by me after a lot of experimention and trial and error!

Dandruff, or, the shedding of dead cells from the scalp can, if ignored, cause acne and minor boils. In the worst case, dandruff, if it spreads to the eyebrows or eyelashes may cause weak eyesight. If your hair is dandruff ridden, it's important to shampoo it every alternate day, rinsing, finally with vinegar and clear running water. Comb your hair daily with a clean comb with rounded teeth. Don't brush wet hair, as this tends to stretch and weaken it. Brush it only when completely dry, starting from the scalp as the sebaceous glands are at the root of each hair. Keep your hair away from your face, shoulders and hands and cut down on soft drinks, coffee and tea; restricting yourself to just herbal teas and drinks. To increase your vitamin B intake switch to cod liver or vegetable oil instead of butter or animal fats. An effective remedy against dandruff is an egg, mixed in 1/2 cup of yogurt applied 30 minutes before shampooing.

Also check for split ends. Hair is made of three layers, the cuticle, the cortex and the medulla. Strong dyes, chemicals, heat, and chlorine can separate these layers causing them to split. Split ends are easily remedied with this treatment: Dip the split ends in a pack of warm olive oil containing 1/2 teaspoon honey. Rub hair lightly. Leave the pack on for 30 minutes. Olive oil nourishes the hair while honey smooths the ends.

If you need to dye your hair use henna; our grandmothers have been using it as a natural hair colorant for centuries. Mixed with yogurt, henna works just as a conditioner, giving your hair bounce and gloss. However, for colour highlights, henna is best used with black tea. Henna can be used to treat oily hair too -- just mix it with coffee, leave it on for 15 minutes, and wash it off. The yolk of an egg and brandy, enlivens dull, lifeless hair, polishing it to a high gloss.

How do you tackle facial hair? Not with regular bleaching, I hope! Bleaching once a month is fine, more often dehydrates. Try this natural bleach: make a mask of crushed strawberries sieved through a muslin cloth. Mix it with an equal proportion of buttermilk. Dab it on. Leave it for 20 - 30 minutes. Don't rinse it with soap; use plain water instead. This treatment can be repeated as often as necessary.

Your hair is a vital beauty asset, requiring tender loving care. Lush, luxuriant, glossy hair is not hard to come by. All it requires is a little nurturing!

Conditioners

I'd recommend these conditioners to anyone whose hair is dull, lifeless or dry. Normal hair too, bounces with added gloss and vitality if you use conditioner after every shampoo.

1 egg, 4 tsp. castor oil, 1 tsp glycerine and 1 tsp vinegar, beaten well till nice and frothy, then worked into the scalp; left for 30 minutes and shampooed off works wonders for damaged hair.

Premature Balding and falling hair:

The finest remedy for this is massaging the scalp with bone marrow. Melt the marrow and massage this oil into the scalp. This oil stimulates growth. Repeat the treatment twice weekly for three months and watch the results!

Specially formulated Oil

200 gms. coconut oil, 25 gms. fenugreek seeds, 2 tsps. henna powder or leaves, 100 gms. green, grated pumpkin. Soak these ingredients overnight. Cook on a slow fire the next morning for 15 minutes, or till the pumpkin turns dark brown and hard. Strain and store. Use this oil only on a clean, dry, scalp. Throw hair forward and brush. With your fingers, apply the warmed oil, gently working it into your scalp. Leave overnight, wearing a scarf or a shower cap to produce body heat that enables oil to penetrate easily. You could even steam your hair with a towel before using this oil.

Treat Those Problems

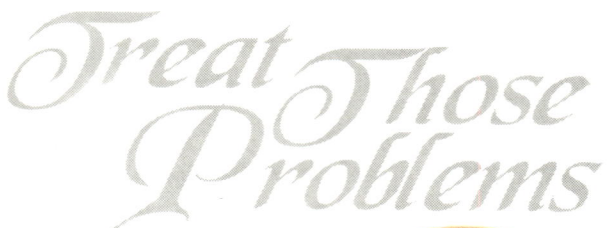

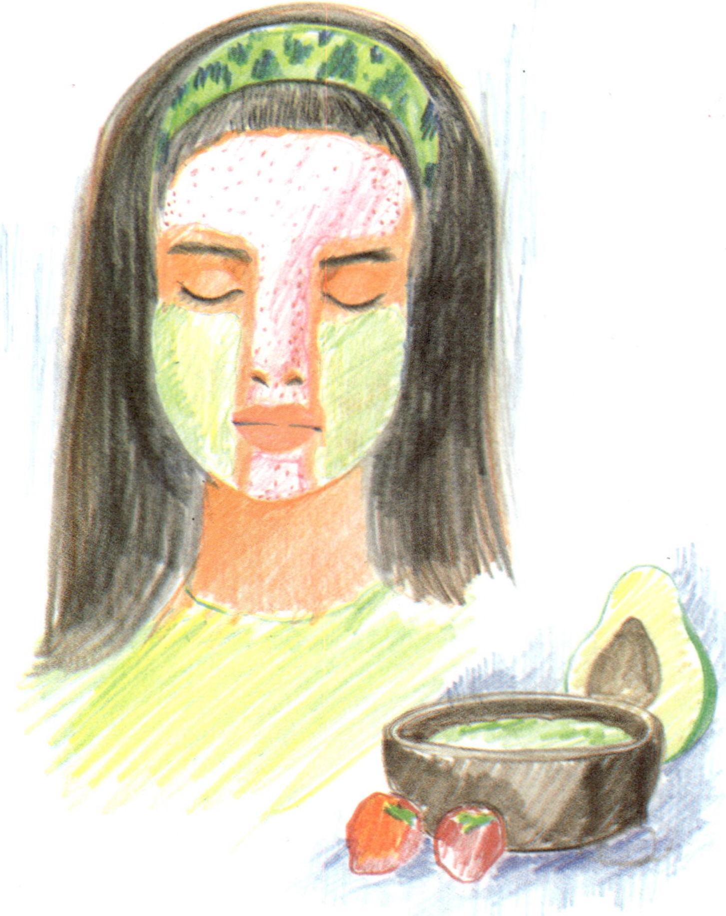

Some consider masks a luxury. I consider them essential as, besides cleansing and beautifying, they relax and restore. They also heal, nourish, boost circulation, tone, iron out wrinkles, freshen, and are, in sum, a fantastic pick-me-up!

The French essayist, Montaigne said: "there is no torture a woman wouldn't endure to enhance her beauty." Thankfully, masks, far from being torture, are magical. This instant skin rejuvenation treatment makes you look younger and fresher in minutes!

Kitchen foods make great masks. You eat food to provide vitamins, minerals and energy. Applied directly on your face, they do the same, enhancing and illuminating your skin.

Masks, incidentally, are the third stage in a facial. In the first stage, the skin is cleansed and steamed to extract blackheads and whiteheads which block the pores and prevent the skin from breathing. Blocked pores cause skin disorders like pimples, acne and sallowness.

The second stage is the toning. Here, the skin is massaged to boost blood circulation, aid absorption of creams and refine skin texture. The warmth generated by the movement of hands dilates the tiny blood vessels that feed the surface layers of the skin, boosting the supply of oxygen and micro-nutrients (vitamins, minerals etc), that the skin needs for it's health. The massage is also a relaxant.

The third stage is the face pack or mask that revitalises skin and improves skin condition. Face packs are always followed by ice pack and astringent treatments to close pores.

I have my own favorite 'pet' masks. After you've tried mine and experimented a little, you'll develop some preferences yourself. My favorites remain those with a base of milk, yogurt and fruit juices. Milk and yogurt are excellent cleansers and refine the pores to boot. The juices get 'soaked' by the skin, providing it with vitamins and minerals. In this chapter, I've described, for easy reference, a range of masks and treatments targeted to different problems. Some of these might have already been included in the preceding chapters.

A rule of thumb: never be in a hurry... pull down the blinds, switch on your favorite music, and relax with your mask, in a darkened room....

MILK MASKS NORMAL/DRY SKIN

The open secret of Cleopatra's famed beauty was milk. She would cleanse her body and her face with milk, and luxuriate in a bath tub filled with this beauty potion. Masks and treatments using milk and other diary products are, by far, my favorite too. Most milk masks are restricted to skins that are normal or dry.

Buttermilk is a great cleanser. Dabbed on cotton and patted on your face, it helps close pores. Leave for 10 minutes and then wash with cold water. Hard to get rid off freckles can be lightened by the daily use of buttermilk patted on, left for 30 minutes, and then rinsed off with cold water.

Cream rubbed, during the cold on chapped or cracked feet and drying skin, left for a while and rinsed off with lukewarm water, will keep your body and face always shining and supple through the coldest winter!

Eggs are one of the oldest beauty aids. The white tones and tightens the skin, while the yolk nourishes and enriches. Stage artists cover their facial lines by applying egg white evenly with a paint brush over the wrinkled area. After the mask dries they use make-up over it. This helps their skin look younger and smoother.

Treat your hair with Eggs too. Massage the yellow of an egg into your scalp-this will stimulate the scalp, giving your hair a special shine. The white has a conditioning effect. Mix in a mug of water and spread over hair. Comb hair in straight strokes and leave for a few minutes before rinsing off with cool water. You'll see a never before manageability and straightness to your hair.

Yogurt cools, smoothens and refreshes. Use all over your body, leave it to dry and take a cool shower. Your body will feel silken to the touch.

Yogurt is especially good for a scaling skin that's dull and gray. It leaves your skin always tingling.

SOME NATURAL REMEDIES

I've listed masks and treatments for every type of skin and problem. It's important to remember though that, in their preparation, mix the juices and liquids first and then the powders. If the mask is still runny, add the powders.

LARGE, OPEN, PORES
Pulped strawberries are astringent and reduce open pores.

Tomato pulp, juice or slices applied on open pores and left for 20/25 minutes helps close pores. Do this daily for quick results. The acid in the tomato does the trick.

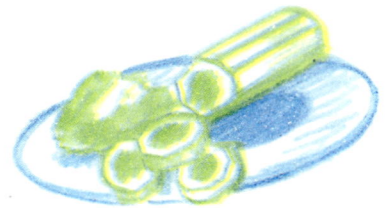

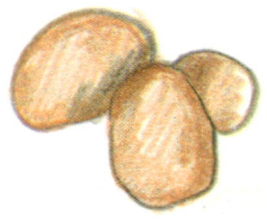

Mix 1 tbsp. yeast grains with enough warm water and allow the mixture to rise. Add 1/4 teaspoon lime juice and a similar quantity of honey. Apply on open pores and leave on for 15 minutes. Repeat at least thrice weekly for results.

A few drops of lemon juice combined with 1 tbsp. of tomato juice applied on open pores for 20 minutes every day helps close pores.

Iced lemon cubes applied daily and allowed to dry on skin shrinks pores.

Dissolve 1 teaspoon bakers yeast in warm water to make a paste. Add 1/2 teaspoon tomato paste and 1/2 teaspoon honey. Apply this paste for 20 minutes on open pores.

OILY SKIN

Thin apple slices reduce oily skin.

Steep 1 tbsp of camomile in 2 tbsp. of hot water and leave for 10 minutes. Strain off. Mix the camomile liquid with oats to make a paste. Add 1/2 a tsp. of honey. Apply twice weekly.

Dab lime juice diluted in water every day on skin.

Tomato slices rubbed on skin daily reduce oiliness.

Rub lemon juice ice - cubes daily on oily skin and leave it to dry for 10 minutes. Great for closing pores and reducing oiliness!

Make a creamy paste with 1 tbsp. grated cucumber, 4 drops lime juice, 1/2 tsp. honey and some oats powder. Apply on oily skin and leave till crisp and dry. Rinse with cold water.

Buttermilk, dabbed on skin for 15 minutes seems to soak up oil.

Strawberry pulp is effective against oil.

1 tbsp. Brewers Yeast tablets mixed with enough yogurt makes a good pack for oily skin.

1 tbsp. low fat milk powder mixed with enough tomato paste to make a paste seems to cut oil. Containing both Vitamin C and Potassium, this pack is a good healer. Use carrot or cucumber pulp if tomato isn't available.

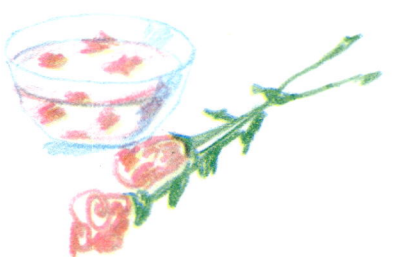

TO LIGHTEN OR FADE TAN

Strawberries, pulped, and spread on cleansed skin.

Cucumber grated, pulped, or sliced, applied on clean skin.

Tomatoes, cut into thin slices and scrubbed onto skin. Leave the juice on for 20-25 minutes, so the acid content of the tomatoes does the trick.

Mix orange peel, sun-dried and pounded into powder, with milk. Leave this paste on your skin for 25 minutes. Rinse off. Do daily for 'lightening' results !

Potato, scrubbed over dark or pigmented skin daily fades pigmented areas.

1 tbsp. powdered almond mixed with a sufficient amount of milk and a pinch of turmeric, if applied daily on wet skin in lieu of soap is an effective bleach.

1 tbsp. soya bean powder mixed with enough curds makes a creamy bleach mask.

Mix equal quantities of Cucumber and tomato paste. Add to almond powder. Use at least thrice weekly. Almonds can be substituted with milk powder.

1 tsp. lime juice and 1 tsp. cucumber juice mixed with a pinch of turmeric powder lightens tan.

SKIN WHITENERS

Each of the following whiteners can be left on the face for at least 15 minutes:

Vinegar

Potato Juice

Cucumber Juice

Lime Juice

Buttermilk

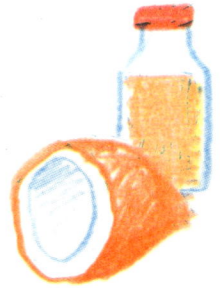

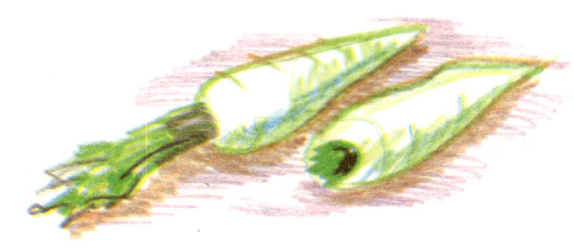

SCRUBS

To make a scrub, add milk, yogurt or orange juice to one of the ingredients listed below:

Green gram powder

Black gram powder

Rice Powder

Almond Powder

WRINKLES

1 tsp. rice or arrowroot starch smoothened on the lines for 20 minutes along with 1/2 tsp. honey help smoothen wrinkles.

SKIN AND BODY COOLANTS

Cucumber is cooling for both skin and eyes. Place cucumber slices, cut round, on your eyes, and grated or pulped on your face. Leave for 15 - 20 minutes.

Camomile tea bags or cotton soaked in camomile tea is extremely cooling.

Rose water and witch hazel mixed in equal proportion and dabbed on your eyes is refreshing and tightening for both skin and eyes.

A soda water wash once a week is a cool, cool freshener!

COMBINATION SKIN

Generally, where your skin is dry, use the treatment for dry skin, and where oily, use the treatment for oily skin.

1 tsp. well beaten egg with 2 drops lime juice mixed with oats on the greasy 'T' area. Then mix a little gelatin with cream and apply to dry areas.

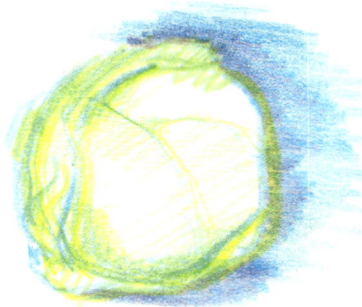

SUMMER TREATMENTS
1 tbsp. egg white and 1 tbsp. yogurt mixed with 1 tsp. lemon juice.

1 tbsp. oatmeal, 1 tbsp. egg yolk, 1/2 tsp. milk and 1 tsp. lemon juice is effective in combating oily skin. 1 tbsp. tomato juice or tomato pulp and 4 drops lemon juice dabbed with cottonwool cuts oil.

A tbsp. oatmeal, one of yogurt and 1 tsp. lemon juice, mixed and applied to dry areas.

DRY SKIN
Avocado is an amazing fruit. Mashed, apply it on dry skin for at least 20 minutes, thrice weekly. Or, add 1 tsp. of lemon juice and one tsp. of egg white to 1 tbsp. of mashed avocado. While removing this mask, add 1 tsp. of salt or sugar. Salt and sugar, being gritty, have an exfoliating effect.

Milk is an excellent cleanser for dry skin. Leave it on for 5 minutes and rinse off with clear water.

Mashed, ripe bananas help smoothen lines and wrinkles on dry skin.

1 tsp. carrot juice and 1 tsp. honey, mixed well with cream is a natural moisturiser if left on the face for 20 minutes; about 4 times a week.

A couple of cod liver oil capsules daily help reduce oiliness.

Warm 1 tsp. of olive oil and 1/2 tsp of glycerine along with a drop of lime juice. Apply a thin layer on dry skin. You could substitute olive with Vitamin E or Almond oil. In winter, this is effective when left on for 10 minutes, and followed by a warm shower without using soap.

1 tbsp. sour cream mixed with a capsule of Vitamin E oil makes a good mask.

Mayonnaise is a great moisturiser for dry skin!

Brushing or using a loofah or scrubs benefits dry skin. It lifts the dry coat and help smoothen roughness. Add 1/2 cup sugar to 1/2 cup yogurt and scrub your skin. This stimulates blood circulation and alleviates dryness.

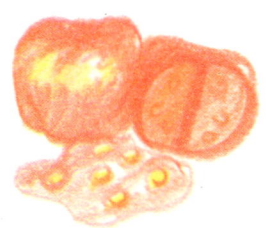 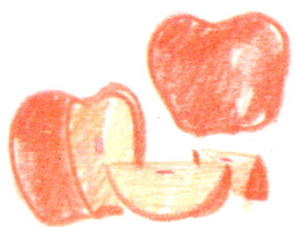

Gently massage a paste of cream and 2 tbsp. almond powder to make a mask. Leave this on your face for 20 minutes.

1 tbsp. egg and 1 tbsp. yogurt mixed with 1 tsp. honey. Apply on face and leave for 15 minutes.

Whip together a mask of 1 tbsp. oatmeal, 1 tsp. yolk, 1/2 tsp. milk and 1/2 tsp. honey.

1/2 tsp. Brewers Yeast, 1 tbsp. honey, 1/2 tsp. vinegar, and 1 tsp. each of sour cream, egg yolk and milk makes a great mask.

Use 1/4 tsp. avocado, 1 tbsp. egg yolk 1/2 tsp. honey and 1/2 tsp. cooking or olive oil to combat dryness.

Combine 1 tbsp. potato pulp with 1/2 tbsp. curds.

Blend together 2 tsp. olive oil, 1 tsp. castor oil, 1 tsp. glycerine and 2 drops lime juice or vinegar and apply on face and hands. After 15 minutes, use a steam towel, finally rinsing with cool water.

Combine 1 tsp. each of cream, egg, powdered milk, honey and powdered masoor dal.

A SCRUB FOR DRY, SCALY SKIN

Take some raw papaya and mix it a with 1 cup of rice powder. This sloughs off dry scales.

WINTER PACKS

1 tbsp. milk powder, 1 tbsp. almond powder, 2 tbsp. glycerine, 1 tbsp. lemon juice, and 1 tbsp. almond or Vitamin E oil is a nourishing winter pack.

1 tsp. vinegar, 1 tsp. glycerine, 1 tsp. almond oil, 1 tsp. Vitamin E oil and 1 tsp. olive oil rubbed well on body and rinsed off after 10 minutes helps counter winter dryness.

A tbsp. cream combined with a tsp. of honey and olive oil, applied on face and left for 20 minutes is a great winter moisturiser.

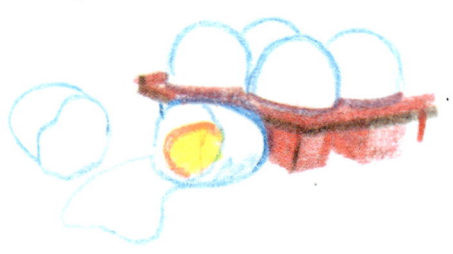

SENSITIVE SKIN

1/2 a tsp carrot juice or pulp combined with 1/4 tsp. honey.

Avocado pulp is soothing to sensitive skin.

Camomile tea dabbed on with cottonwool. Leave on for 5 minutes.

Cod Liver oil, too, has a soothing effect.

Cucumber juice or pulp is soothing.

A combine of 1/2 vinegar and 1/2 water, soothes, when dabbed on skin.

Spread a tsp. of plain yogurt evenly on face.

Dab cottonwool dipped in mint tea on your face; leave on for 7 minutes and rinse off with cool water.

1 tbsp. cream and 1 tsp. honey soothes sensitive skin.

WARTS

Warts drop off if Vitamin E oil is applied on them daily.

Cauliflower juice, left on warts overnight, wears them out.

Chip the top of a garlic clove and apply on the warts. Leave the garlic juice on overnight.

FRECKLES

Freckles lighten by using buttermilk on them daily for 20 minutes.

Radish juice applied daily lightens freckles.

Powdered almonds with strawberry pulp and cream lightens freckles.

Potato slices rubbed on freckles lightens them.

Tomato slices also lighten freckles.

1 tsp. milk powder and lime juice diluted with water makes a quick, whitening pack for freckles.

Rub cucumber slices daily to lighten freckles.

Vitamin E oil applied daily on freckles helps lighten them.

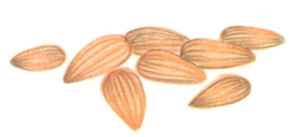
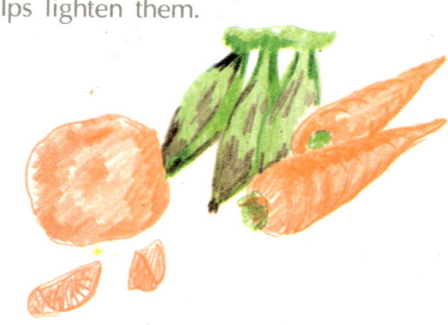

CHAPPED FACE & CRACKED AREAS DURING WINTER

Rub milk cream on the affected area and leave it on for 30 minutes before showering. This will help your skin remain supple and shining.

Rub the green skin of watermelon on cracks.

A glycerine and lime combination helps lessen cracks.

For itchy feet, rub onion juice between toes; or rub the wet onion well on the area. It reduces itchiness.

UNDER EYES PUFFINESS

Grate raw potato or place thin slices of potato on puffy eyes. I find potato juice on cotton eyepads placed over puffy eyes helpful. Keep your head raised on two pillows.

Use cotton pads soaked in equal quantities of rosewater and witchhazel to reduce puffiness. If your skin is very dry under the eyes, use a thin film of Vitamin E oil before placing the cool eye pads. Have in stock 10 - 15 soaked, refrigerated eye-pads always.

Soak 2 pieces of round cotton pads in cold milk. Place this over your eyes. Place two pillows under your head to drain off puffiness.

BLEMISHED SKIN

Carrot Juice, applied daily, fades blemishes. In fact, carrots, rich in vitamins A and C, are excellent for skin disorders.

Watermelon juice, left for 15 minutes on the face helps clear blemishes.

Coconut Oil massaged on blemished skin every night lessens marks. Vitamin E oil, too, helps lessen marks.

Rub tomato slices on blemishes daily. Leave on for at least 15 minutes.

Strawberries and raw potato are natural lighteners.

1/2 tsp. of honey and 1/2 tsp. of yogurt, mixed well with almond powder makes a smooth paste. Leave it on for 20 minutes every day.

Dab coconut water on blemishes and leave it on for at least 10 minutes.

Radish, spinach, parsley and potato juice are individually effective in lessening blemishes, when applied on skin daily.

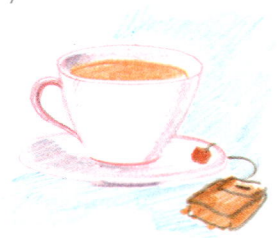

SCRUBS FOR DEAD CELLS AND LUSTERLESS SKIN

Pineapple, if crushed and applied on the face for 20 minutes helps to slough off dead cells.

Oats, sugar and rice powder, blended separately with Yogurt, have the same effect.

A papaya mask rids the skin of dead cells and impurities. My mother tutored me to tenderise the toughest meat by adding pieces of papaya. I merely added this to my mask collection! Cover your well scrubbed face with a muslin cloth spread with mashed papaya. Rinse after 20 minutes. Now watch it glow!

Scrub 1 tbsp of red lentil powder with 1/2 tsp. of honey and enough rosewater to make a smooth paste. Apply on skin. Leave it on for 5 minutes; then, scrub it off. This helps remove dead skin. If your skin is very dry, mix warm milk with almond powder and mashed avocado or almond oil. Being soft, it won't hurt if you rub this into your skin vigorously.

SLUGGISH, DULL SKIN

Grated cucumber in muslin, left on eyes and face helps revitalise skin. The silicon and sulphur content in cucumber peps tires skin.

I love Brewers Yeast for it's special quality of coaxing blood to the skin's surface, giving you a healthy glow. Taken internally, Brewers yeast powder keeps both hair and skin shiny. A warning: use a yeast mask at least 3-4 hours before you go out, as the pep in blood circulation might cause your skin to get warm and flushed. This mask is a combine of 1 tbsp. Brewers Yeast, 1/2 tsp yogurt and 1/2 tsp honey. The honey and yogurt should be mixed first.

Strawberry works as an astringent, lightener and toner. It's enzymes help tone a tired, dull skin, reducing the oils and refining the pores.

Combine 1/2 a tsp of egg yolk with 1/2 tsp of lemon juice and olive oil. Slowly add cornflower to make a creamy pack. Apply with brush or fingers. Leave till taut and dry. Follow up a luke warm rinse with a cool rinse.

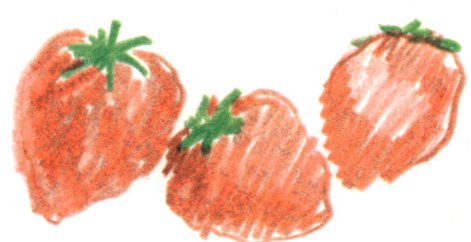

Combine 1 tbsp Cucumber, 1 tbsp. egg white, some milk powder and 1 tsp. brewers yeast to make a paste. Wash off after a while.

BLACKHEADS

Foment you face (after cleaning) with a steamed towel that was soaked in water containing 2 tbsp soda bicarbonate. Change the steam napkin 6-7 times. Now use a gentle scrub - try 1 tsp. yogurt and 1 tsp. rice powder. The blackheads, loosened by the steaming, will fall off. Always, as a finale, follow a steaming session with a cold water rinse to close pores and discourage blackheads.

PIMPLES

Grated carrots, pears or their juice helps disinfect and soothe the skin.

1 tbsp. of ripe, mashed banana is excellent for pimply skin. You may add 1 tsp. of rice powder to scrub the pack off after 15 minutes.

Brewers Yeast mixed with low fat yogurt makes a creamy paste that activates the skin besides cleaning the pores of grime.

Tamarind is a cooling, antiseptic that reduces skin oils. A paste of tamarind applied thrice a week prevents pimples.

A mint paste mixed with yogurt and oats powder is an excellent cure. Leave it on for 20 minutes daily.

Mash 1 tsp. grated cucumber into a pulp. Add enough low fat powdered milk and a tsp. of egg white to make a paste. Apply this to the pimpled areas, leaving on for at least 15 to 20 minutes.

Cabbage, being acidic, helps cure pimples. You can pulp the cabbage, and with a gauze, leave it on the skin for 20 to 30 minutes thrice a week.

FOR PEDICURES AND MANICURES

Bathe feet and hands in warm water with 2 lids vinegar and 1 tbsp lime juice added, along with a bit of body shampoo. This keeps hands and feet smooth.

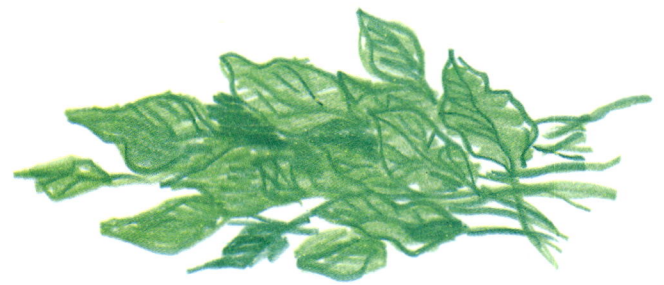

TO TONE AND TIGHTEN SKIN
Apply egg white twice a week.

A mask of mashed ripe banana, kept on face for 20 minutes and rinsed off with cold water firms the skin. Do this every other day for good results.

Mix 1/2 tsp. of honey and 3 Vitamin E capsules with cornflour to make a paste and apply to a well scrubbed face and neck for 20 minutes. Rinse off with cold water. This is great for crows feet.

Apply 3 capsules of warmed Vitamin E oil on the face concentrating on the lines. Then spread well beaten, frothy egg white in upward direction. Leave till it dries. Rinse off with cold water. Then moisturise.

1 tsp. carrot paste mixed with 1/2 tsp. honey and 1/2 tsp. castor oil spread on lines for 20 minutes is a good wrinkle treatment.

1 tbsp egg white mixed with 1/2 tsp. honey and enough milk powder to make a smooth paste. This should be applied in an upward direction.

Strawberries and cream also make a great mask. Mix it in equal proportions.

ROUGH PALMS
1 tbsp. sugar and 1 tbsp. any oil scrubbed well on palms softens them.

SUNBURN
Mint Paste is cooling and lightening.

Yogurt or buttermilk will soothen or lighten.

Potato Pulp is soothing.

Coconut juice is cooling.

Sunburn can be cured by dabbing cotton in cool tea and applying on the sunburn. Leave it for 20 minutes.

DARK UNDERARMS AND NECK
Apply lemon juice and a pinch of turmeric mixed with cucumber juice for 20 minutes daily. This should cure you of this problem.

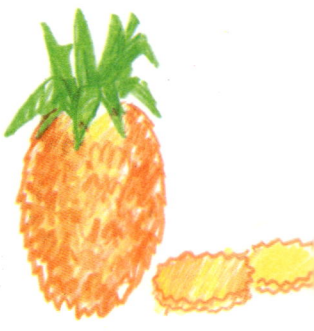

DULL, DAMAGED HAIR

Egg massaged into your hair is a stimulant, giving your hair a special sheen.

Steam towel your hair. After 2-3 minutes massage a mixture of an egg and 1/2 a cup of yogurt. Increase the quantities of both depending on the length of hair. Shampoo after 25 minutes, wrapping up with a vinegar rinse.

A final rinse of 2 tbsp. vinegar to a tumbler of cool water gives a lovely sheen to your hair.

DARK CIRCLES UNDER EYES

The most effective treatment is ... soak 1/4 kg almonds in milk overnight. Peel the next morning and grind the almonds with milk to make a paste. For the pack, use 1 tbsp. paste with 3 drops lemon juice. Place on eyes for 30 minutes. Refrigerate the remaining almond paste and use every day as mentioned.

Grated potato makes a great eye pack.

Tomato paste smeared under the eyes is effective in lightening circles.

Vitamin E oil dabbed under your eyes helps alleviate the problem.

Cucumber slices, cut round and placed on each eye.

Apple slices placed over each eye helps lighten dark rings.

HAIR CONDITIONER FOR BOUNCE AND GLOSS

1/2 a cup of vinegar and 2 cups of water left on hair for five minutes and rinsed, gives your hair bounce and gloss.

For dry hair try 1 tbsp. glycerine and 1/2 cup cider vinegar in a tumbler of water. Leave on scalp for 15 minutes. Rinse off using a light shampoo.

Mix egg white in a mug of water and spread over well shampooed, rinsed hair. Comb hair in straight strokes and leave for some minutes before rinsing with cool water. You'll notice your hair gets extra body and looks well conditioned.

Mash ripe avocado and spread on hair, massaging thoroughly for 15 - 20 minutes. Then rinse.

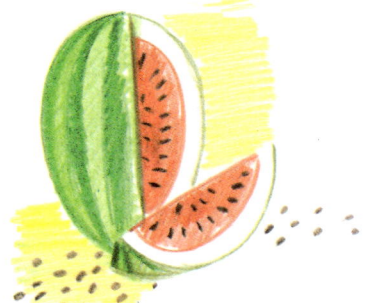

DANDRUFF

Apply 4 tsp. of warm olive oil mixed with 1 1/2 tsp lemon juice. The next day, make a pack of 1 egg and 1 tbsp yogurt. Leave on scalp for 30 minutes. Rinse off shampoo and finally rinse with a tumbler of water with 3 lids vinegar.

Apply 1/2 cup of yogurt and 1 egg mixed well with Brewers yeast powder. Apply on scalp. Allow for an hour to dry. Shampoo off, finally rinsing with vinegar.

2 tbsp glycerine and 1 tbsp lemon juice combined with 1 tbsp. coconut oil. Mix vigorously. Apply this on clean, dry hair. Keep on scalp for 1 1/2 to 2 hours. Steam your hair with warm towels 5 - 6 times. Shampoo off with egg shampoo.

2 tbsp. of lemon juice in a tumbler of water, as a final rinse after shampoo reduces dandruff. After about 5 minutes, rinse out with cool, clear, water.

FALLING HAIR

A warm oil massage with this recipe handed down to me by my mother really helps: 200 gms. coconut oil, 25 gms. powdered fenugreek seeds, 100 gms grated, green pumpkin, and 2 tbsp. castor oil. Soak these ingredients overnight. The next day, cook them on a slow fire till the pumpkin turns brown. Strain and store. Always massage oil by using cotton dipped in warm oil on a clean scalp. Shampoo with egg shampoo and finally rinse with 4 lids of vinegar diluted with a tumbler full of water.

Bone marrow massaged into your scalp at least 3 times a day helps to reduce falling hair. If you can leave this on overnight, there's nothing like it, but even a couple of hours helps.

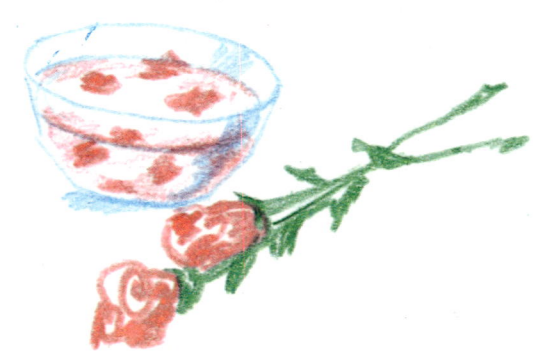

Your Questions... Answered

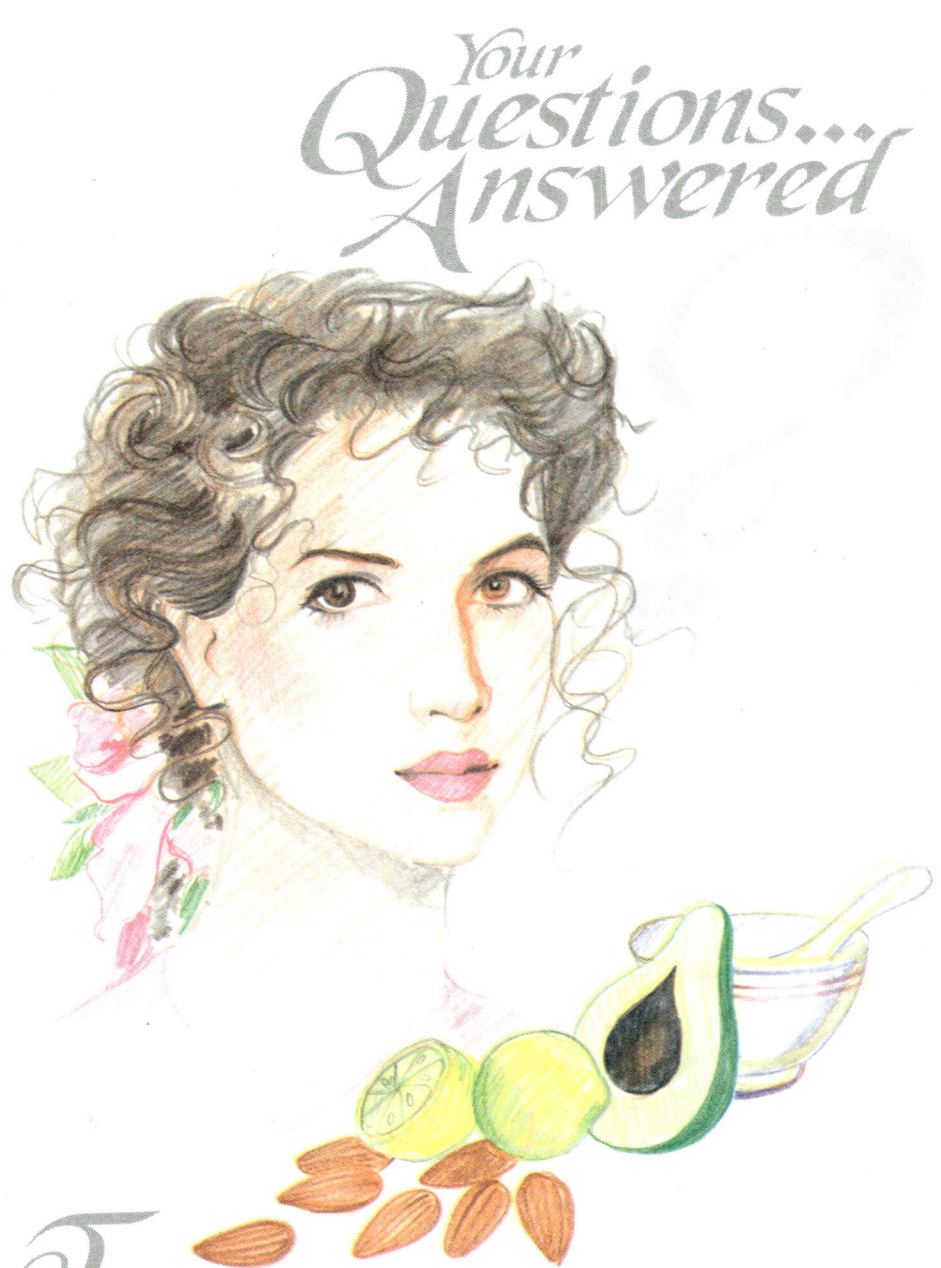

These are everyone's favorite questions. I have given just one treatment for each question. For others, do refer to the relevant chapters, or the relevant subheads in the chapter: " Treat those Problems".

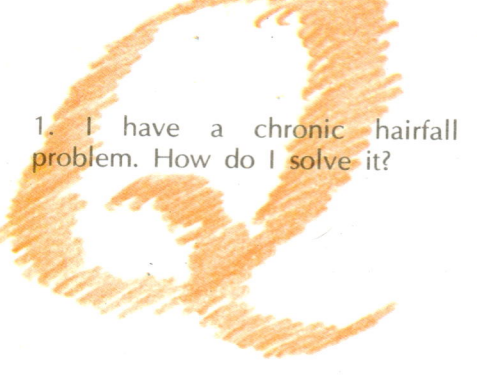

1. I have a chronic hairfall problem. How do I solve it?

Recipe: Soak the following ingredients overnight: 200 gms. coconut oil, 25 gms. methi (fenugreek) seed powder, 100 gms. grated green pumpkin, 2 tbsp. castor oil. Soak all these overnight. The next day cook on a low flame till the pumpkin gets light brown. Cool and strain. Massage your scalp when clean at least 3 times a week using either a cling film, cap or steam towel to allow oil to penetrate the pores. Shampoo, finally rinsing with 4 lids vinegar in a tumbler of water.

2. How do I lighten my tan?

Treatment: Rub a slice of tomato immediately after you come in from the sun. Leave the juice on for 20 minutes; then rinse.

3. I have large, open pores. How do I remedy this?

Recipe: Blend 1 tsp. tomato juice, with 2 drops of lime juice and 1/4 tsp. honey. Leave this on your skin for 20 minutes every alternate day. Rinse off with cold water.

4. How do I soothe tired eyes?

Treatment: Apply cool tea or camomile tea bags on your eyes daily, for 10 minutes.

5. What is an effective skin cooler in warm weather?

Treatment: Plain yogurt left on skin for just 15 minutes and rinsed off with mint tea water works wonders.

6. How do I treat warts?

Treatment: A little cauliflower juice applied on warts helps them drop off gradually.

7. My skin is always tired and dry. How can I make it glow?

Mask: 1 tbsp. strawberry pulp with 1 tbsp. almond powder works wonders when blended and applied on face for 20 minutes. Scrub off with cold water.

8. How do I cure acne?

Mask: Blend 1 tbsp. crushed mint with enough oats powder. Leave the mask on your face for at least 20 minutes. This reduces pimples.

9. How do I enliven a dead, dull skin?

Mask: Combine 1 tbsp. egg yolk with 1/2 tsp. honey, 1 tsp. olive oil, and 2 drops lemon juice and enough almond powder to make a creamy paste. Apply on face. Remove once the mask firms by rinsing with cold water.

10. My skin is dry. How do I remedy this?

Treatment: Combine 1 tsp. glycerine, 2 drops lime, 1/2 tsp. olive oil, 1/2 tsp. vinegar. Massage this on your face, leaving it for five minutes. Rinse off with cold water.

11. How do I reduce blemishes?

Treatment: Apply carrot juice on blemishes daily, leaving it on for 20 minutes.

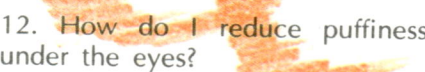

12. How do I reduce puffiness under the eyes?

Treatment: Dip round cotton pads in cold milk and rest on eyes for 10 minutes. Place 2 pillows under the neck to drain off the puffiness.

13. How do I lighten freckles?

Treatment: Buttermilk applied daily helps lighten freckles. It must be left on for not less than 15 minutes.

14. My face and feet are chapped.

Treatment: Blend 1 tsp. glycerine with 2 drops lime juice and 2 drops oil (cooking, almond, olive or Vitamin E). Apply this daily leaving it on overnight.

It rejuvenates your skin instantly.

15. My skin has a tendency to sag. How do I firm it?

Mask: Apply a ripe, mashed banana on your face for 20 minutes daily.

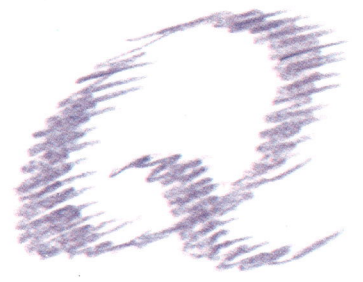

16. How do I nourish my skin?

Mask: 1 tbsp. honey and 1 tbsp. yogurt makes an effective, creamy mask. Left on for 20 minutes, it rejuvenates your skin instantly.

17. My palms are rough. How do I soften them?

Treatment: Use a mixture of 100 ml. glycerine and 1 tsp. lime juice. Prepare this in advance, shaking the bottle before using on palms.

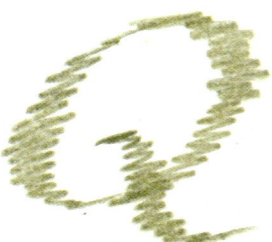

18. How do I repair dull, damaged hair?

Treatment: 1 tbsp. castor oil combined with 1 tbsp. honey and 1 egg yolk massaged onto scalp before rinsing is therapeutic on damaged hair.

19. How do I add body to limp hair?

Treatment: Beat an egg white stiff and mix in a tumbler of water. Use this as a conditioner. Rinse with cool water.

20. How do I alleviate sunburn?

Treatment: Apply yogurt on affected areas.

21. How do I alleviate dandruff?

Treatment: Combine 2 tbsp. glycerine, 1 tbsp. lemon juice, 1 tbsp. castor oil and 2 tbsp. fenugreek seed powder with 1 tbsp. vinegar. Massage this onto scalp and leave for 30 minutes. Rinse off with cool water.

22. How do I smoothen and soften my hands and feet?

Treatment: Warm water in basin with 2 caps vinegar and 1 tbsp. lime juice. Add a little baby shampoo. Dip hands and feet for 10 minutes, finally rinsing with cold water.

23. I have an oily skin. What can I do?

Treatment: Thin apple slices rubbed onto skin help reduce oiliness.

24. How do I reduce dark circles under the eyes?

Treatment: Tie potato pulp in muslin and rest on eyes for at least 10 minutes daily. Use a light film of oil or cream after you have removed the mask as this may cause dryness.

25. How do I lighten dark underarms and neck?

Treatment: Apply 1 tbsp. cucumber juice combined with 2 drops lime juice and a pinch of turmeric on dark areas for 20 minutes daily. This is a natural bleach.

26. How do I cure pigmentation?

Treatment: Apply coconut oil daily on pigmented skin. Leave it overnight on pigmented areas.

27. How do I reduce facial hair?

Treatment: Apply 1 tbsp. egg white blended with 1 tbsp. sugar and enough cornflour to make a sticky paste. After 5 minutes gently lift the peel off pack. Some hair will be removed. For best results, repeat this 3-4 times a week.

28. My scalp is dry and itchy. What can I do?

Treatment: Scrub on scalp 1 tbsp. vinegar and 1 tsp. lime juice. Leave on for 15 minutes before shampooing; then rinse off with cool water.

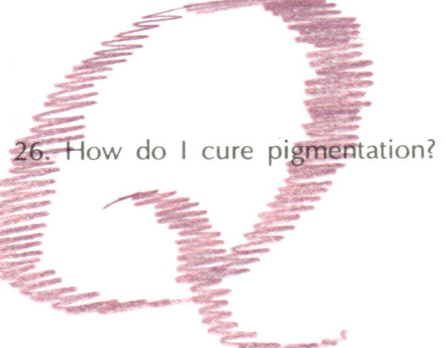

29. My nails are broken. What can I do?

Treatment: Massage the fingers daily with warm oil, pushing back cuticles gently with an orange stick. Include gelatine in your diet at least thrice weekly.

30. What can I do about crows feet?

Treatment: Apply 1 tsp. honey and 1/2 tsp. cream on crows feet Rinse after 20 minutes. If repeated frequently, the crows feet, over time, will smoothen.

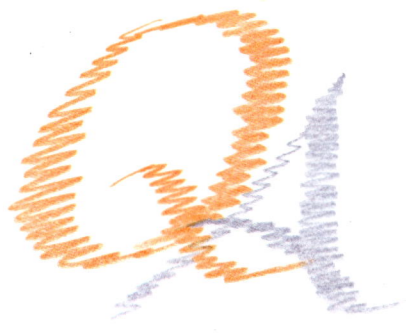

The Finishing Touch

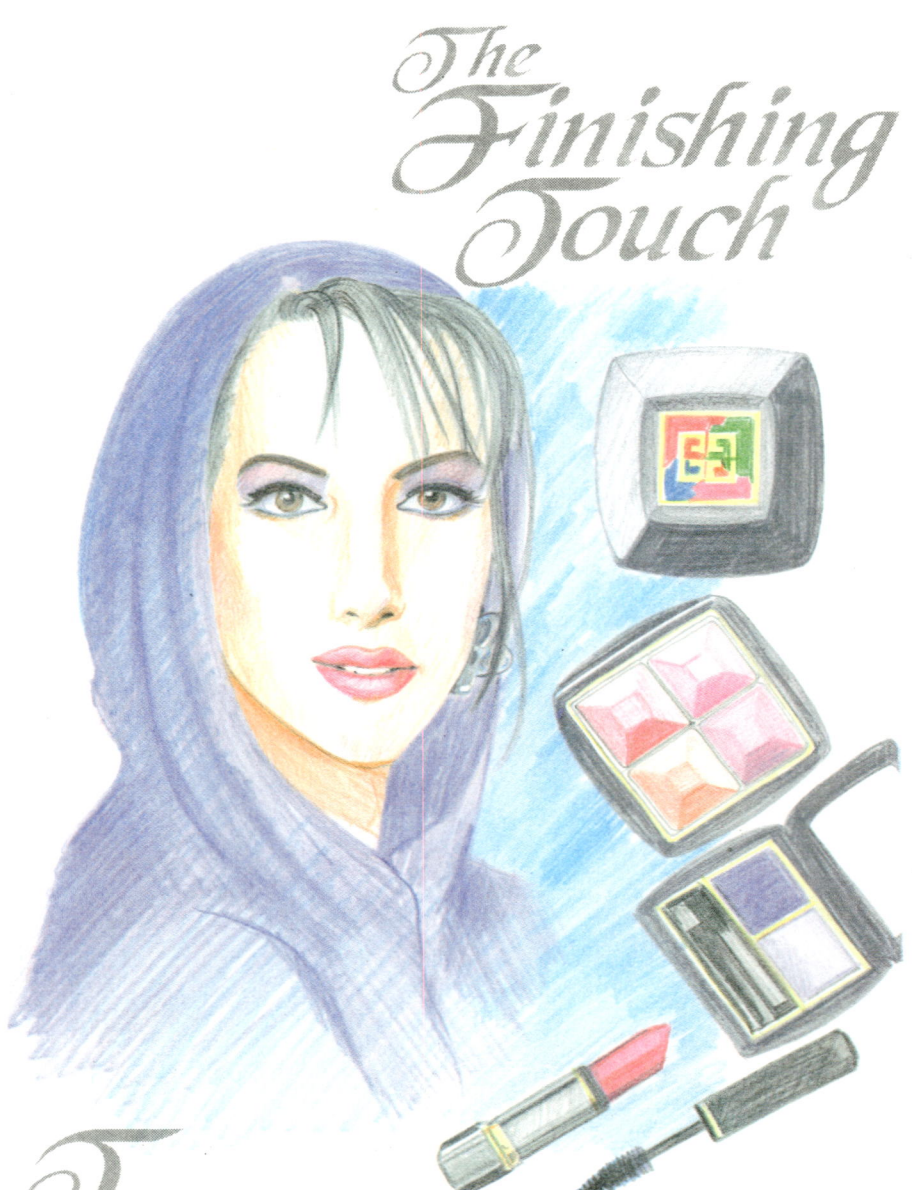

*T*reat your face as you would a canvas. You wouldn't splash it with colours without a definite vision; a definite goal. Your face, your soul's mirror, as it were, certainly deserves to be treated with the same respect!

At the outset, check out your face by pulling your hair back off your face with a headband and examining your features and skin tones. Write down the features you like best and those you're not happy with. Once you 've recognised your pluses and drawbacks, you're in a position of strength. You now know the features you'll highlight and those you'll correct or downplay. Whichever way you play it, follow this golden rule: dark shades reduce the size of your features and light shades bring them out. In applying your make-up, move from one logical step to another.

CLEANSER

Cleanse your skin thoroughly. Tone with a toner or astringent; then moisturise your skin to give it a smooth texture and protect it's natural moisture.

FOUNDATION

Foundation evens out skin tone, improves skin colour and hides minor blemishes giving a smooth texture to your complexion and protecting your skin from weather and the drying effects of central heating. Most women need a light application of foundation; and remember, less is always more -- the more subtle your make-up, the more effective it looks. Foundation is always applied downwards to minimise the impact of facial hair. I personally feel it's more natural to match foundation to skin colour. Always use a damp sponge to apply the foundation covering every part of the face well. Choose the shade by blending it into your jawline rather than your hands and remember to choose it in the daytime. Foundation creates a smooth flawless finish, enabling you to accent your best features.

CONCEALER

Two shades lighter than your skintone, concealer corrects make up, blemishes, lines on the sides of the mouth, nose, and the inside corner of the eyes. Dark circles can be corrected by applying concealer exactly on the demarcation line between the cheek and the eye and blending it into that very line. Anything else will give you a pouchy look.

POWDER

The purpose of powder is, not to add colour, but to set, and blend make-up. Powder also alleviates the shine on your face.

BLUSHER

A blusher can contour or highlight, depending on how its applied. The ideal place to apply blusher is right below the cheek bone starting from the corner of the iris and going towards the ear and up towards the temple. Blusher adds a healthy glow to the complexion.

EYES

These are the hardest features to work with. Eye make, the most popular of all make up, should never be rushed, as the smallest of errors have a tremendous impact. Make up your eyes in 3 steps:

CANVAS: The canvas, which is eyeshadow colours that echo skin tones, i.e. beige, pink, peach, and coral goes on the entire eye area, from the corner of the nose right till the corner of the eyes.

CONTOUR: Contours, the opposite of canvas, darken and create illusion by combining shading and highlighting techniques.

A rule of thumb: canvas pushes in while contouring brings out. You contour with neutral shades, using greys, brown and charcoal. Choose your contour shades by matching it to your hair colour, so that you stay within the boundaries of your natural skin palette.

ACCENT: These are the brilliant hues: blue, green, purple and violet. Apply accent on both eye corners. And instead of matching your accent to your eye colour, use a contrast: ie, with blue eyes try green turquoise, combine black eyes with purple and slate eyes with violet or purple.

LINER: You could use this under or on top of the lid. Liners are liquid or pencil. If your eyes water whilst applying liner make a tissue in a slim pencil point and just touch the inner corner of your eyes to reduce tears.

MASCARA: Always apply mascara to bottom lashes first. Allow it to dry and repeat the coat to thicken.

LIPSTICK

I use a two tone theory on lips. Your base tone is a neutral brown or beige. Use this like a canvas. Cover the entire lip with this. Outline your lips to give the right shape. Fill in the lipstick colour with a brush. Finally, apply a hint of gloss. You're now all set to go! But wait a minute...spray your face first with Evian or Rosewater spray or prepare your own spray by mixing 1/2 witch hazel and 1/2 water. Spray sets the make up and leaves skin looking fresh for hours.

SOME MAKE-UP TIPS

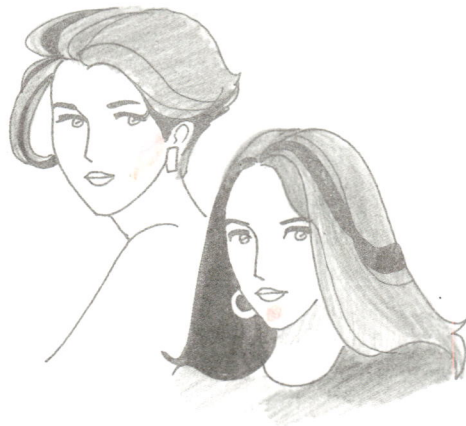

TO GIVE A HIGH CHEEK BONE EFFECT

1. Apply the blusher under the cheek bone in the hollow going towards the outer ear towards temples.

2. Apply a very light shade on the bone area to give a cheek bone effect. You may apply a little blusher to the nose, forehead and chin.

TO SHORTEN A LONG FACE

1. Apply the blusher into the hollow of the cheek blending up to the sides.

2. Avoid the blusher on temples.

3. Apply lightly on forehead to distract the length of the face and apply a hint on the chin to reduce length.

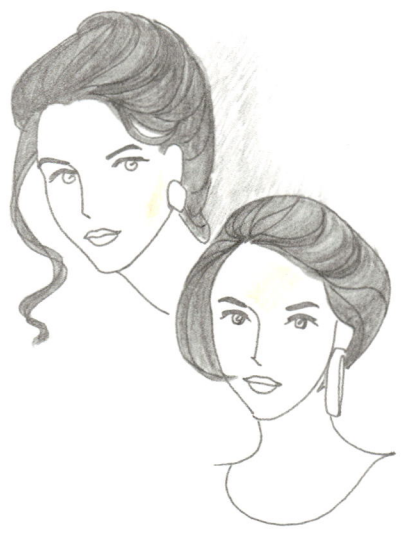

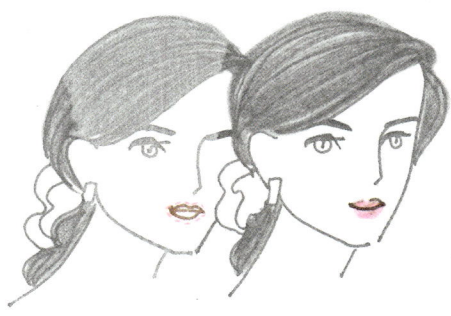

IMPROVING THIN LIPS

1. Apply the lip pencil outside natural lip line.

2. Apply a foundation on the lips extending it upto the newly created lip line.

3. Using a light lip colour, apply your lipstick right upto the new lip line.

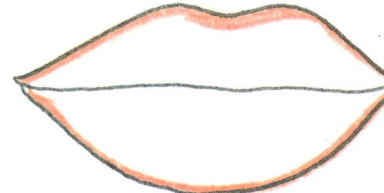

REDUCING THICK LIPS

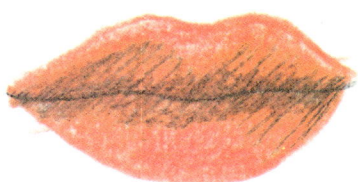

1. Use the lip pencil inside natural lip line.

2. Apply a foundation on the lips and dab loose powder. This helps the lips look thinner.

3. Use dark shades to reduce fullness.

SHAPING SHAPELESS LIPS.

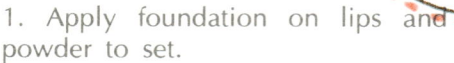

1. Apply foundation on lips and powder to set.

2. Using the lip pencil use the pencil on the outside natural lip line for the thin lips.

3. Where the lips are thick use a lip pencil in the inside of the lipline.

4. Use light lipstick on the thin lips and dark on thicker lips. The contrast should be slight.

TO WIDEN CLOSE SET EYES

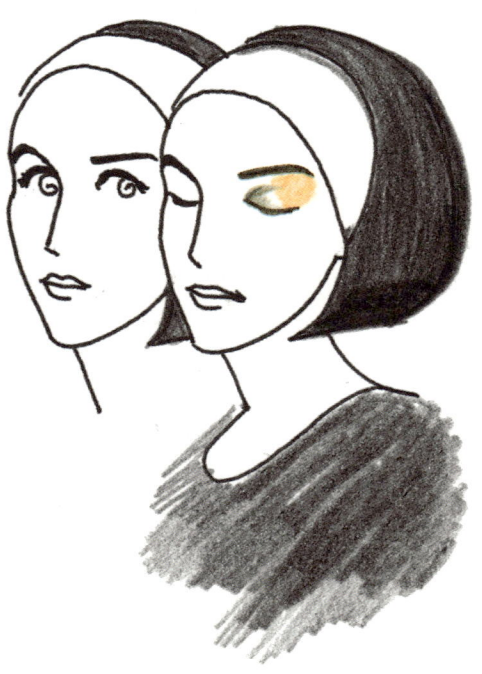

1. Use the light shade from your eye compact in the inner corner of the eye lid, covering only half the lid towards the centre of the lid.

2. Now the dark tone should be applied on the outer corner of eyes. This gives an elongated look.

3. Blend the 2 colours lightly.

4. The dark tone is blended from the middle of lid upwards to the brow bone extending beyond the outer corners of the eyes.

5. The highlight is used under the brow.

6. Eyeliner is used away from the corner of the eyes on the top and lower lids.

ENLARGING SMALL EYES

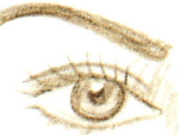

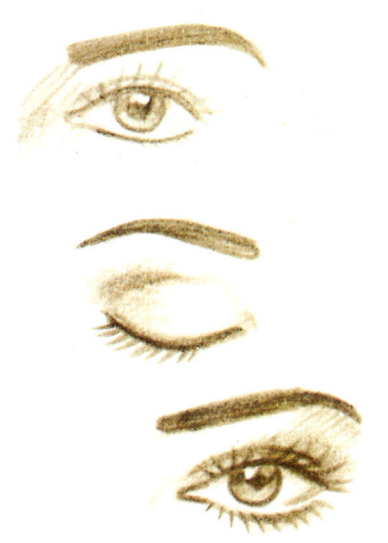

1. The outer corner of the eyes require a medium tone eye shadow, shaped upwards.

2. The dark colour is applied on the eye crease.

3. The medium shadow is used on the entire eyelid.

4. Apply the highlight below the brow.

5. The eyeliner on the upper lid should be from the inner corner to the outer corner. Start the liner on the lower lid from about 1/3 of the eye towards outer corner.

WIDE-SET EYES

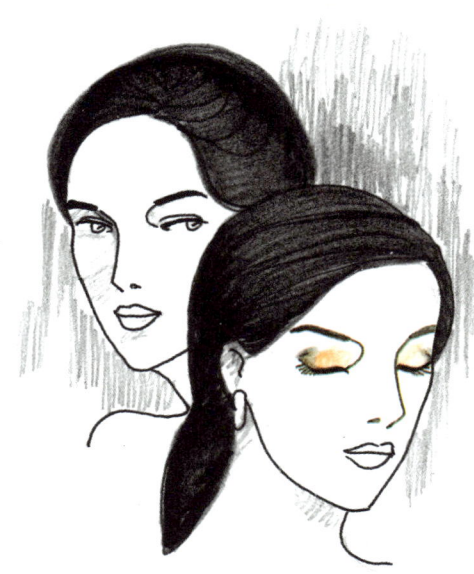

1. A medium tone shadow is used and worked towards the outer corner of the eye. This gives a slanted, upward look.

2. While applying the shadow angle it upwards at the corner of the eye and blend well.

3. The corner of the eyes need a dark shadow. Work softly along side of the nose into the full area of the brow. Always blend well.

4. Work the lightest shadow into the centre exactly under the brow.

5. Line the eye on the upperlid only moving from the eye corner to outside the vicinity of the eye area. Use a brown shadow line on lower lid.

6. Line the lower lid just a little away from the corner of the eye moving towards the end of the eye.

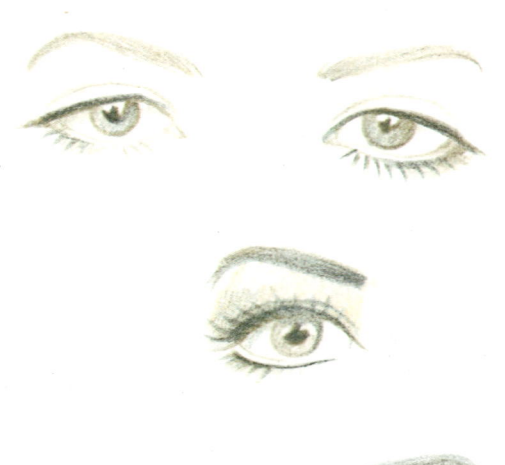

DROOPING EYES

1. Lift droopy eye by applying eye shadow in an angle on the outside.

2. Use upward strokes to lift the eyes.

3. Blend a lighter shade into corner of eyelid blending, again, upwards following the sides of the nose right upto the brow.

4. Apply a dark shade in the centre crease of the brow bone.

5. The upper liner should stop at least .a little before going to the corner. Leave at least one eighth from the outer corner unlined .

6. Line 3/4 of the lower lid starting from the outer corner.

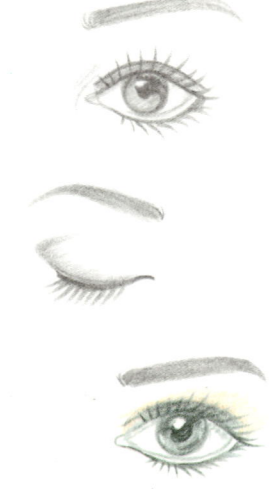

DEEP SET EYES.

1. Apply a medium toned shadow at a slight angle on the outer eye corner.

2. Use a medium light shade on the entire eyelid, blending softly into the brow bone.

3. To open eyes blend a light shade in the centre of the eyelid.

4. Never use dark shadow near brow as this will make your eyes appear even more deep set. Use, instead a light shadow.

5. Never use eyeliner.

THIN EYEBROWS NEED THICKENING.

1. The eyebrow should begin parallel to the inner corner of the eye and end just beyond the outer corner.

2. The eyebrow should be fullest at the nose bridge and softly taper at the end in line with the eye corner.

3. Use a brown or taupe pencil to colours brows. Black will reduce size further.

4. Powder brow with brown and use a mascara brush to brush against and towards the brow. This adds fullness. You can then comb to tidy them.

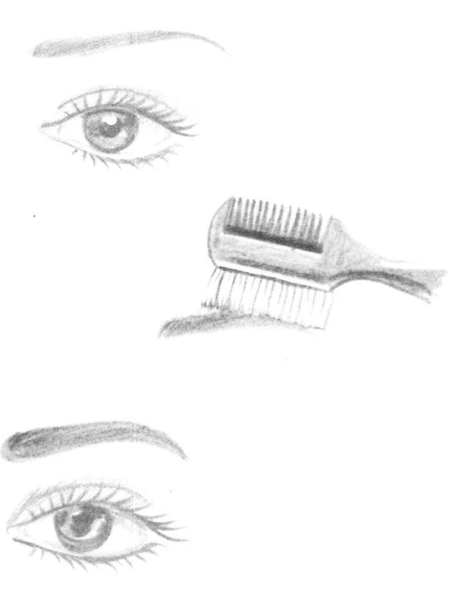

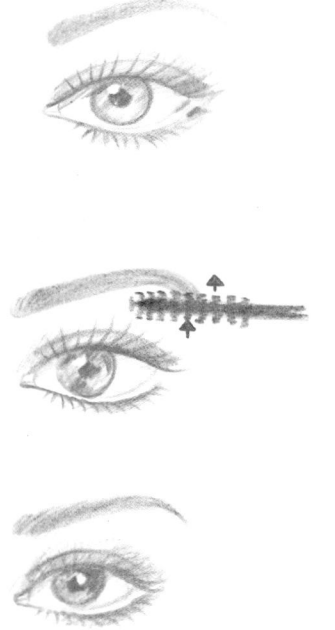

SPARSE EYEBROWS NEED THICKNESS

1. Use a brown eye shadow pencil to colour brow.

2. Don't change their natural shape.

3. The eyebrow should begin parallel with the inner corner of the eye and end just beyond the eye.

4. The strokes should be gentle. You could even draw in individual hairs between your natural hairs.

5. Use the eyebrow brush to fill in colour and brush.

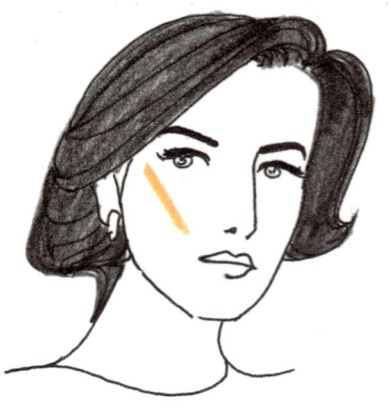

TO EMPHASISE HIGH CHEEK BONES

1. Use a blusher two shades darker than your skin shade.

2. Draw a line under cheek bone in the hollow of the cheek starting in line with the corner of the iris and moving out towards the ear

3. Blend the shade. The darker, remaining in the hollow. Don't forget to blend the line.

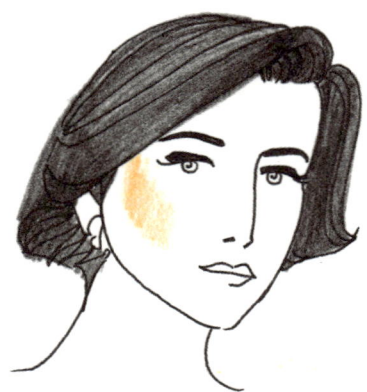

EXTEND A BROAD NOSE

1. Apply dark colour on either side of the nose bridge in a straight line.

2. If the nostrils are wide you need to entend the line down towards the end of nostrils.

3. You must avoid the center of the nose bridge.

4. Blend softly always.

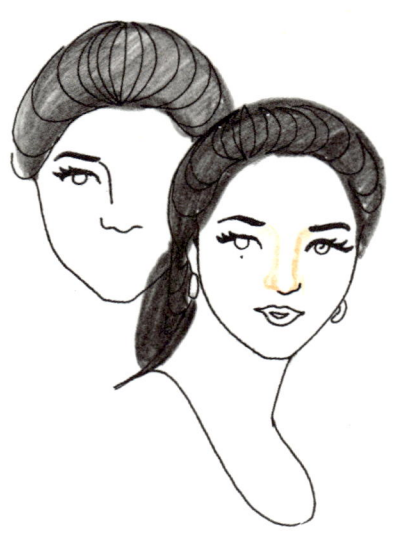

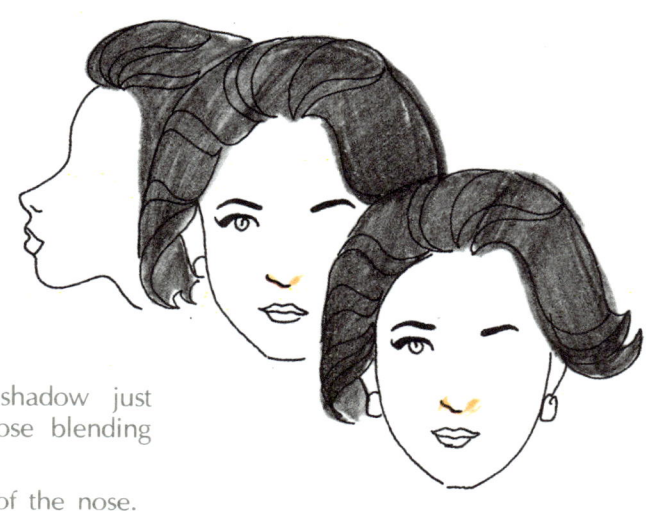

TO SHORTEN A LONG NOSE

1. Apply a darker shadow just under the tip of the nose blending around half the nostril.

2. Don't colour the tip of the nose.

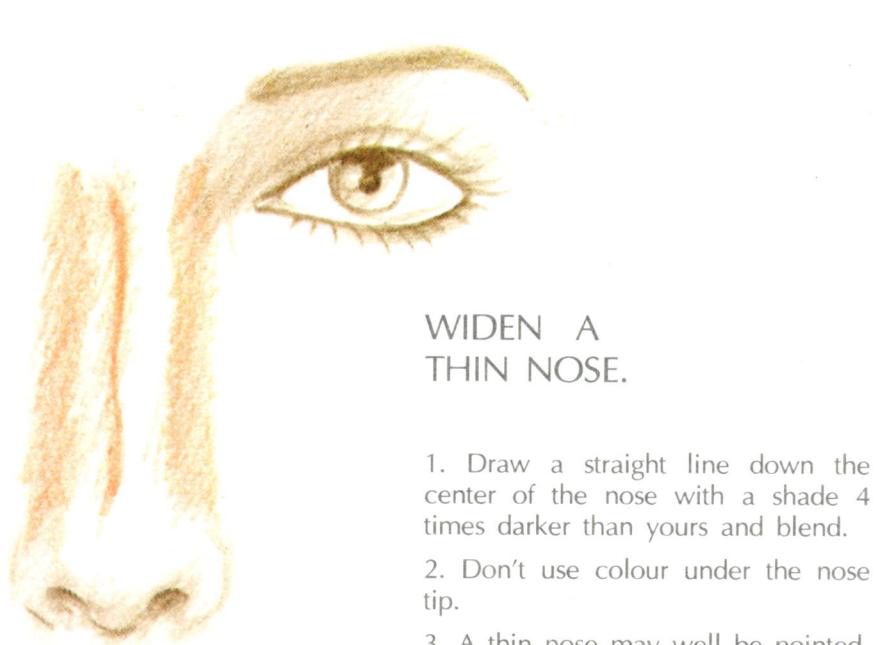

WIDEN A THIN NOSE.

1. Draw a straight line down the center of the nose with a shade 4 times darker than yours and blend.

2. Don't use colour under the nose tip.

3. A thin nose may well be pointed. The dark line going down from the centre of the nose should be just till the tip of the nose - not under.

About the Author

Rima Soni, born and brought up in Bombay, trained in beauty care in London and New York. She has been a practising beauty consultant since 1978. Her beauty treatments, gleaned from across the world, combine the best of Eastern and Western thought.

Rima lectures in schools, colleges, clubs and associations, apart from the beauty demonstrations she has conducted for Avon and Lakmé in the UAE. She is well known in Dubai and the U.A.E. for her beauty columns in *Gulf News*, *Khaleej Times*, *International Indian* and *Telelife*. Rima Soni has given a new meaning to the title: Kitchen Cosmetologist!

Inspite of having resided overseas for over a decade, Rima's heart belongs to India. This book is a tribute to her country.